THE
KIDNEYS
& URINARY
SYSTEM

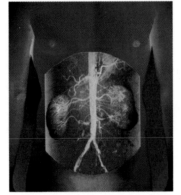

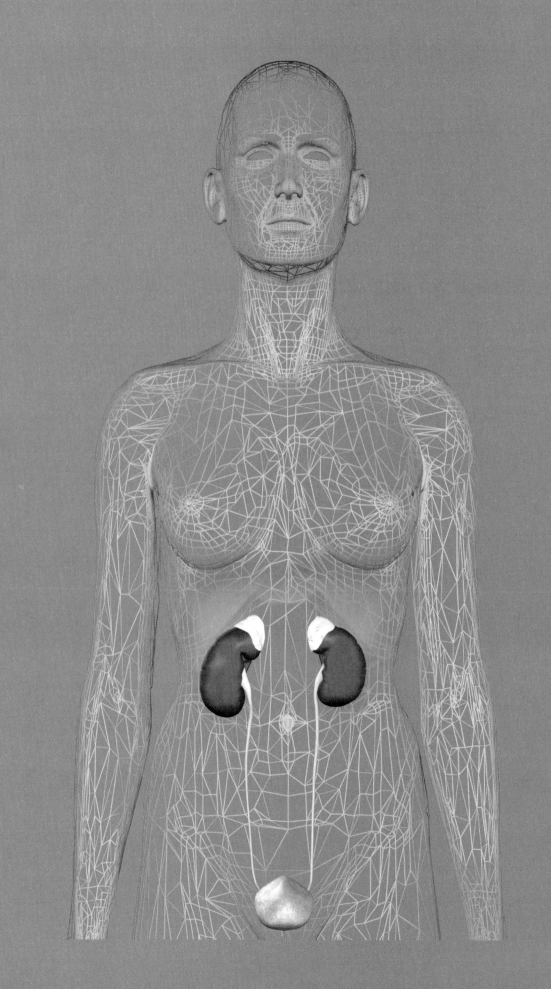

THE
KIDNEYS
& URINARY
SYSTEM

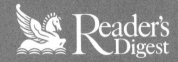 Reader's Digest

The Reader's Digest Association Limited
London New York Sydney Montreal

The Kidneys and Urinary System

was created and produced by
Carroll & Brown Limited
20 Lonsdale Road
London NW6 6RD
for Reader's Digest, London

First English Edition Copyright © 2002
The Reader's Digest Association Limited
11 Westferry Circus
Canary Wharf
London E14 4HE
www.readersdigest.co.uk

Copyright © 2002 The Reader's Digest
Association Far East Limited
Philippines copyright © 2002 The Reader's
Digest Association Far East Limited

ISBN 0 276 42702 5

Reproduced by Colourscan, Singapore
Printed and bound by Printer Industria
Gráfica S. A., Barcelona

The information in this book is for reference only; it is not intended as a substitute for a doctor's diagnosis and care. The editors urge anyone with continuing medical problems or symptoms to consult a doctor.

Managing editor
Anne Yelland

Managing art editor
Anne Fisher

Editors
Judy Fovargue, Marianne Canty, Anna Southgate

Art editors
Maxine Lea, Vimit Punater

Design assistant
Justin Ford

Series medical consultant
Dr Lesley Hickin, MB BS, BSc, DRCOG, MRCGP, General Practitioner

Nephrology specialist consultant
Professor Stephen Huw Powis, BSc (Hons), BM, BCh, PhD, FRCP, Director, Centre for Nephrology, Royal Free and University College Medical School, University College London, and Head of Department of Nephrology and Transplantation, Royal Free Hospital, London

CONTRIBUTORS

Dr Aine Burns, MD, FRCP, Consultant Nephrologist and Honorary Senior Lecturer, Centre for Nephrology, Royal Free and University College Medical Schools, London

Dr James Balmforth, BSc, MB BS, MRCOG, Clinical Fellow in Urogynaecology, Kings College Hospital, London

Wynnie Chan, BSc, PhD, Public Health Nutritionist

Michael D. Dinneen, MD, FRCSI (Urol), Consultant Urological Surgeon, Chelsea and Westminster Hospital, London

Chrissie Gallagher-Mundy, BA (Hons), Fitness Writer, Director, London Academy of Personal Fitness

Katy Glynne, BSc, MRPharmS, Dip Pharmacy Practice, Clinical Services Manager, Charing Cross Hospital, London, Clinical Lecturer, The School of Pharmacy, University of London

Dr Ed Kingdon, MB BS, MRCP, Nephrology Specialist Registrar, Royal Free Hospital, London

M.E.J. Lean, MA, MD, FRCP, Professor of Human Nutrition, University of Glasgow, Consultant Physician, Glasgow Royal Infirmary

Miss Rachel Busuttil Leaver, BSc (Hons), RN, Clinical Nurse Specialist for Continent Urinary Diversions, Middlesex Hospital (UCL Hospitals Trust), London

Joel Levy, BSc, MA, Medical Writer

Professor Stephen Huw Powis

Dr Paul Sweny, MA, MB, BChir, FRCP, MD, Consultant Nephrologist, Royal Free Hospital, London

Dr David Wheeler, MD, FRCS, Senior Lecturer in Nephrology, Royal Free Campus, University College, London

For Reader's Digest
Series Editor Christine Noble
Art Editor Julie Bennett
Editorial Assistant Lucy Murray
Reader's Digest General Books
Editorial Director Cortina Butler
Art Director Nick Clark

The Kidneys and Urinary System

Awareness of health issues and expectations of medicine are greater today than ever before. A long and healthy life has come to be looked on as not so much a matter of luck but as almost a right. However, as our knowledge of health and the causes of disease has grown, it has become increasingly clear that health is something that we can all influence, for better or worse, through choices we make in our lives. *Your Body Your Health* is designed to help you make the right choices to make the most of your health potential. Each volume in the series focuses on a different physiological system of the body, explaining what it does and how it works. There is a wealth of advice and health tips on diet, exercise and lifestyle factors, as well as the health checks you can expect throughout life. You will find out what can go wrong and what can be done about it, and learn from people's real-life experiences of diagnosis and treatment. Finally, there is a detailed A to Z index of the major conditions which can affect the system. The series builds into a complete user's manual for the care and maintenance of the entire body.

This volume zooms in on the kidneys and urinary system, showing how these structures control the levels of fluid in the body and fine-tune the balance of salts and other chemicals in the body's cells. See what goes on inside the tiny filtering units that form the basis of the kidneys' complex refining processes, constantly working to eliminate substances that could be harmful. Learn how to assess what is normal for your own kidneys and bladder, how healthy bathroom habits are key to maintaining these organs, and how medications, food and drink, exercise and even clothes can affect your urinary health. Find out about the body's fluid balance and the optimum water intake not just for kidney health but for general well-being. And discover what can threaten the health of the urinary system, how problems are diagnosed and identified, and the medical, surgical and practical treatment options available for dealing with kidney and urinary diseases and any other problems that can arise.

Contents

3

What happens when things go wrong

The life story of the kidneys

The urinary system might not be the most glamorous part of the body, but in practice the kidneys and their associated plumbing make up one of the most important body systems. They constitute a biological water treatment and waste disposal system of great sophistication and enormous capacity, whose functions directly affect the health and very survival of every cell in the body.

Life evolved in the oceans as loose assortments of biomolecules that were extremely vulnerable to changing environmental conditions. A great evolutionary leap occurred when these loose assortments began to surround themselves with membranes, giving rise to the first cells. Each of these cells was like a tiny enclosed fragment of the ocean, a drop of salty liquid in which the biomolecules could operate — with one huge difference: the cell membranes isolated the internal environment of the cell from the outside world, preserving stable conditions in which the machinery of life could function efficiently.

As evolution progressed and life forms became more complex, involving precise and delicate interactions between thousands of different molecules, so the need to preserve stable internal conditions became even more important. Many of the organs and body systems of higher animals are devoted to just this end, a process known as 'homeostasis' — the maintenance of a constant internal environment.

WATER, WATER, EVERYWHERE

This is where the kidneys and urinary system come in. As in those first, primitive cells, our internal environment resembles the ocean — it is mostly water, with many different dissolved salt ions. The amount of water and the precise concentrations of these different salts must be maintained within very narrow parameters or the cells of the body will not function properly, and will soon die. But there are many factors at work that threaten to upset the balance of water and dissolved salts in our bodies.

The simple life
The first life forms were simple organisms, such as Closperidium — loose accumulations of salt water ions in an enclosing membrane. Although infinitely more complex, the body's cells similarly rely on everything being in balance, which depends on regulation by the kidneys.

Humans cannot survive without access to fresh water: the kidneys cannot process the salt in seawater – we would die from dehydration if we had to rely on it for drinking.

Water and salts enter our bodies when we eat and drink, and are lost as we breathe and sweat. The biochemical processes of cell metabolism create a range of waste products, including water and dissolved substances such as urea, which not only upset the delicate balance of our body fluids but can be toxic is they are allowed to if they are allowed to accumulate.

What the body needs is a system that can minutely regulate the composition of the body fluids while at the same time extracting and disposing of the waste products of metabolism. This system is, of course, the urinary system made up of the kidneys – which process body fluids (in the form of blood) and produce urine to dispose of metabolic waste products and excess water and salts – and the bladder and urinary tract, which transport, store and eliminate urine. The system also includes a series of control mechanisms that monitor the composition of body fluids and adjust kidney function accordingly. The adrenal glands, which sit on top of the kidneys, play a role in these control mechanisms, as well as producing hormones that help to control other body systems.

PUNCHING ABOVE THEIR WEIGHT

Kidneys are present in all vertebrate life forms, from the most primitive to the most complex, but it is in the higher vertebrates such as humans that they have reached the peak of sophistication. Your kidneys combine great processing power with adaptability to a wide range of conditions and extreme precision. For instance, despite making up just 0.4 per cent of total body weight they receive almost a quarter of the blood pumped out by your heart, and they process the entire volume of blood plasma (the fluid in which red blood cells float) 60 times a day – that's once every 24 minutes! This allows the kidneys to get rid of dangerous or unwanted substances very fast, and gives them rapid and powerful control over the volume and composition of the blood plasma, and by extension all body fluids.

The amount and concentration of urine that they produce can vary enormously to meet the most extreme environmental challenges. For instance, if your body needs to expel salts they can produce urine that is four times more concentrated than your body fluids, whereas if you need to conserve salts, they can produce urine that is just one sixth as concentrated as your body fluids. The daily volume of urine that they generate can be as low as 0.5 litres, or as high as 20 litres.

PRESSURE CONTROL

By controlling salt and water levels in blood plasma, your kidneys also control blood pressure, protecting you against dangerous increases (which give rise to a condition known as hypertension) that might result from excessive

Urination in utero
This ultrasound shows a baby boy urinating in the womb. Urine in the urethra is coloured blue, turning red/blue as it leaves the penis and comes into contract with amniotic fluid.

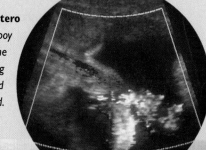

consumption of salt. In the developed world, levels of dietary salt average ten times higher than is needed for homeostasis. Fortunately, your kidneys are so good at their job that a 50-fold increase in salt intake causes only a minor rise in blood pressure.

Your kidneys have other abilities too. They filter out and excrete acids produced during protein metabolism, including sulphuric and phosphoric acid. They regulate vitamin D production, converting it from an inactive to an active form. They can even generate glucose, the sugar that your body uses as an energy source, if your survival is threatened by starvation. If your kidneys ceased to function you wouldn't survive for long. Within a few days enough water, potassium, acid, urea and other substances would accumulate in your body to kill you.

THE LIFE OF THE KIDNEYS

The kidneys and urinary system are present early in development. They mature through childhood, developing their complexity and tight control, which will continue to serve most people well into old age.

THE LIFE STORY OF THE KIDNEYS AND URINARY SYSTEM

The powerful and sophisticated machinery of the urinary system starts life soon after fertilisation as a line of tissue called the urogenital ridge that runs more or less down the centre of the tiny embryo. What is unusual about the development of the urinary system is that from this point it sets off on a series of false starts before the true kidneys and urinary tract actually form, perhaps representing in developmental terms stages in the evolution of progressively more complex urinary systems.

The first of these false starts, known as the pronephros stage, begins very early, in the 4th week of embryological development. The top of the urogenital ridge forms into a series of tubules that serve no apparent purpose – they never become functional and disintegrate almost as soon as they form, leaving only a pair of ducts that stretch down the back of the embryo.

The second false start comes in the 5th week of development, when tissue further down the urogenital ridge, known as the mesonephros, develops into a series of

about 20 tubules. These tubules get as far as hooking up with offshoots of the aorta, the embryo's main artery, to form large, primitive nephrons – the basic functional units of the kidney – but again these never function and soon degenerate, leaving only the same duct as before, now known as the mesonephric duct.

Finally, at the base of the urogenital ridge, a mass of tissue known as the metanephros begins to form into proper kidneys. Meanwhile, in the wall of each mesonephric duct, ureteric buds form – these are blind-ended tubes that grow into the metanephric tissue and begin to branch. These branches will eventually become the structures that collect urine in the kidneys and feed it into the ureters, the long tubes that carry urine from the kidneys to the bladder.

Although the young kidneys soon start to function in a rudimentary fashion, at this stage there is relatively little for them to do – almost all of the waste produced by a developing baby is removed from its bloodstream

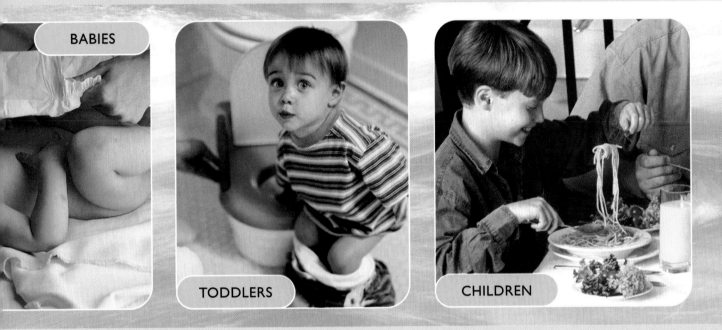

BABIES

TODDLERS

CHILDREN

Learning control
Children differ widely in the age at which they master control of going to the toilet: it depends on maturity of their urinary system, and on their desire and willingness to learn to stay dry.

across the placenta and disposed of by the mother's urinary system. The tiny amounts of urine produced are stored in the cloaca, a primitive combination of anus and urinary outlet, and the allantois, the vestigial human version of a chicken embryo's yolk sac. Near the end of the second month of development the embryo's cloaca subdivides into the rectum and urinary outlets, while the allantois degenerates and disappears, except for its base, which becomes the bladder. The connection between the two is known as the urethra.

BEANIE BABIES

By the end of the third month of development, all the elements of the urinary system are in place and the kidneys have assumed their familiar bean shape. However, they will not be required to function properly until birth, when they have to take over excretory and fluid-balancing duties from the placenta.

After birth the urinary system grows along with the rest of the body. The nephrons continue to develop and become more complex, taking between six months and six years to reach full maturity – some do not become fully mature until the age of twelve. Conscious control of the bladder (known as continence) also takes time to develop, as both the sphincter muscles and the nerve connections needed to operate them are immature at birth.

POWERS OF ADAPTATION

After this the urinary system changes little until late adulthood. The bladder descends slightly at puberty and

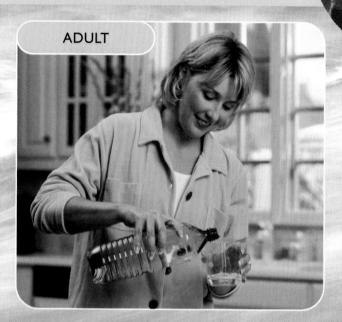

Screen test
In this false colour-enhanced intravenous urogram, the bladder, filled with contrast medium, shows up red. The enlarged prostate can be seen as a gold shadow beneath it.

ADULT

OLDER PEOPLE

Drinking for health
Staying properly hydrated is vital to maintain concentration ability and mental well-being, as well as physical health.

Gland to watch
In males, the prostate naturally enlarges with age. This can have an impact on the ease and frequency of urination in older men, but early awareness can help to avoid serious problems.

the number of nephrons in the kidney starts to fall very gradually from the age of 25. Not until after the age of 40, however, does this decline begin to become significant; beyond this age it is normal to lose ten per cent of your nephrons every ten years. Although this sounds serious – especially since nephrons are unable to regenerate – in practice it has little effect on a healthy urinary system because your kidneys have an astonishing degree of reserve capacity.

You can lose up to 70 per cent – possibly even 80 per cent – of your kidney function before problems set in, thanks to the incredible powers of adaptation possessed by the nephrons, which increase the capacity of the remaining tissue. Individual nephrons can quadruple their efficiency to compensate for the loss of others through kidney damage.

WATER WORKS
This doesn't mean, however, that renal health can be taken for granted. The kidneys and urinary system are absolutely central to overall well-being, and impaired kidney function becomes a particular problem in the context of ill health, when a compromised urinary system can exacerbate other conditions. And the kidneys are vulnerable to some of the most common diseases – leading causes of kidney failure include high blood pressure, diabetes and heart attacks. In 1994, for instance, more than 15 million people in the USA suffered from some form of kidney disease.

This means that a healthy lifestyle that helps you to avoid conditions such as hypertension and diabetes will also help to keep your urinary system in good shape. More specific steps include drinking plenty of water, practising good hygiene and boosting your awareness of age-related

If all the nephrons in the kidneys were laid end to end, they would stretch for about 80km (50 miles).

problems such as enlargement of the prostate (a gland that sits just below the bladder in men), which can affect sphincter function.

KIDNEYS IN SPACE

Medical intervention in the arena of renal health is extremely advanced. Drugs are available to control most aspects of kidney function, and by juggling types and doses doctors can fine-tune treatment regimes. If kidneys fail, advanced dialysis machines can be used to mimic the functions of the urinary system, and although it is hard for even the best devices to match the efficiency of the real thing, thousands of people have survived for 15 to 20 years on dialysis, with good quality of life.

Perhaps in the future we may even see dialysis machines small enough to be implanted, acting as artificial kidney replacements. Other advances are likely to come in the field of drug design, where pharmacologists

are working to overcome one of the natural barriers to the longevity of drug effects – the kidneys' efficiency at removing from the bloodstream substances recognised as artificial in the body.

Genetic engineering offers the prospect of treatments for kidney and urinary tract cancers and hereditary problems, and one day it may even be possible to re-engineer human kidneys to enhance their natural health and endurance. Kidneys could be engineered to be better at removing toxins and pollutants from the bloodstream, for instance, or to be more effective at counteracting high blood pressure. In the far future it may be possible to design a urinary system that would allow its host to live on seawater, or survive on hostile arid planets where water is in short supply. For those of us with a more down-to-earth lifestyle, however, the kidneys and urinary tract provide a better life support system than anything that NASA can devise.

Arid adaptations
Camels are especially suited to desert life, thanks to their fur and fatty hump which prevent body temperature rising to sweating point, the major cause of water loss in other species, including humans. In the future, scientists may be able to modify human kidneys to give humans similar resistance to dehydration, enabling people to live in arid environments..

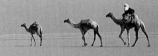

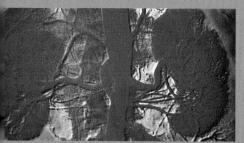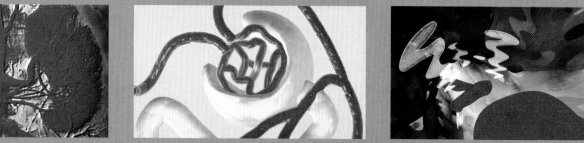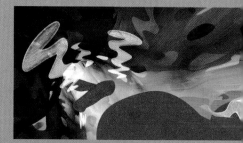

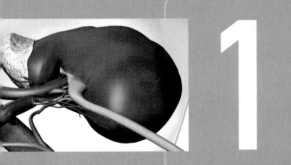

1

How your kidneys work

Your amazing kidneys and urinary system

Your urinary system does more than simply get rid of excess water – it minutely controls the composition of your body's fluids, maintaining the delicate balance essential for life, while at the same time expelling harmful waste products.

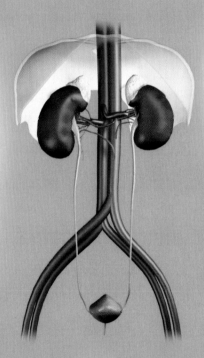

WATER WORKS

The urinary system could be compared in some ways to a sewage works. Both take fluids that are polluted with waste products, clean them and dispose of the waste while returning the cleaned fluid to circulation. But the urinary system is more efficient, complex and capable than any sewage system devised by man. It doesn't simply filter bad stuff out – it actively selects what should go and what should stay. It plays a vital role in regulating blood pressure, and has an important endocrine (hormone-secreting) function. In men, the urinary system also overlaps with the reproductive system, carrying seminal fluids to their destination.

BLOOD AND URINE

The primary function of the urinary system is to make and dispose of urine, a fluid that is 95 per cent water, the remainder being dissolved salts and organic substances. Your body uses urine to dispose of nitrogen-containing waste molecules that are produced by cells as they process proteins and nucleic acids, such as DNA. Whatever doesn't leave in the urine remains in the blood, so that by controlling the composition of urine your kidneys also control the composition of your blood and consequently of the other fluids in your body.

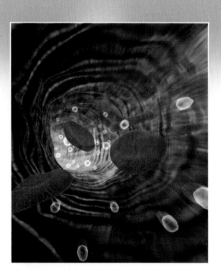

Helter skelter
Get a close-up perspective on the progress of a red blood cell as it passes through the kidney's maze of blood vessels and tubes. See pages 30–31.

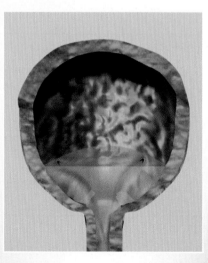

When you gotta go
A combination of hormonal and nervous signalling systems control how much urine you produce and how long you store it before triggering the bladder to empty. Pages 36–37 reveal these processes at work.

Male and female *urinary systems differ in some significant ways. See pages 18–19 and 36–37 for further details on the differences between the sexes.*

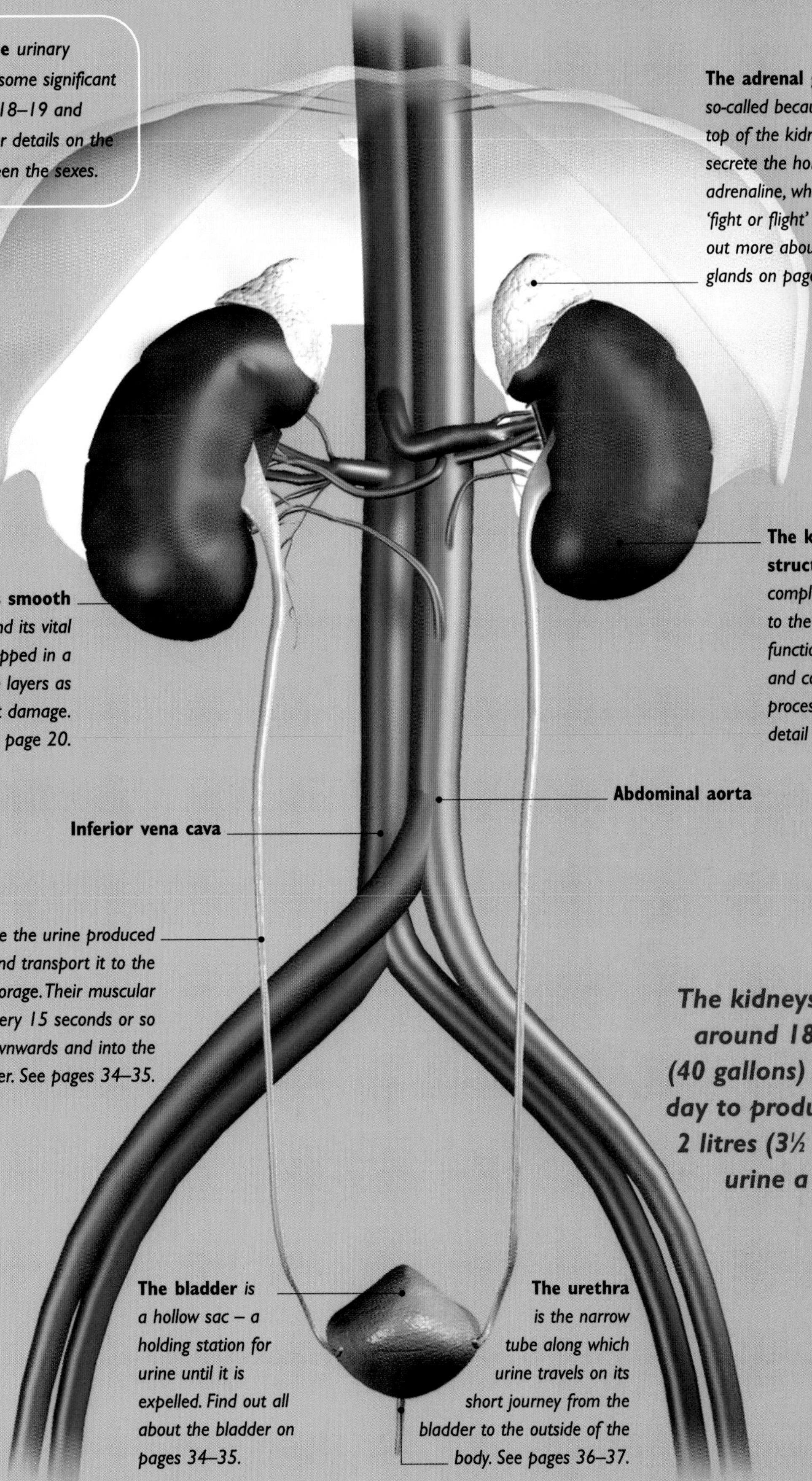

The adrenal glands *are so-called because they sit on top of the kidneys. They secrete the hormone adrenaline, which triggers our 'fight or flight' response. Find out more about these amazing glands on pages 32–33.*

The kidney's internal structure *is highly complex and closely tied to the organ's primary function of producing and collecting urine. This process is explained in detail on pages 22–29.*

The kidney's smooth inner capsule *and its vital contents are wrapped in a series of protective layers as a safeguard against damage. Find out more on page 20.*

Abdominal aorta

Inferior vena cava

The ureters *take the urine produced in the kidneys and transport it to the bladder for storage. Their muscular walls contract every 15 seconds or so to move urine downwards and into the bladder. See pages 34–35.*

The kidneys process around 180 litres (40 gallons) of fluid a day to produce about 2 litres (3½ pints) of urine a day.

The bladder *is a hollow sac – a holding station for urine until it is expelled. Find out all about the bladder on pages 34–35.*

The urethra *is the narrow tube along which urine travels on its short journey from the bladder to the outside of the body. See pages 36–37.*

Locating the urinary system

The different elements of your urinary system are some distance apart, distributed through your abdomen and pelvis. There are some significant differences in the way they are organised in men and women.

BACK TO BACK

The kidneys are positioned on either side of the vertical midline of your body, between the navel and the bottom of the sternum. They sit nearer to your back than your front, behind most of the abdominal organs, and at a slight angle so their front faces are tilted outwards. The kidneys move up and down slightly as you breathe and ride up by about 2.5cm (1in) when you lie down. Between them they make contact with various other organs, including, on the right side, the liver and duodenum, and on the left, the spleen, pancreas, stomach and colon. These organs help to support the kidneys and keep them in place.

The diaphragm separates the chest and abdominal cavities.

The inferior vena cava *carries deoxygenated blood from the parts of the body below the diaphragm – including the kidneys – back towards the heart.*

The right kidney makes an impression in the liver where it squashes up against it. Your right kidney sits slightly lower than your left in order to accommodate the mass of the liver above it.

The abdominal aorta *is the body's largest blood vessel. It travels down the centre of the abdomen carrying oxygen-rich blood. Branches from it feed blood directly to the kidneys.*

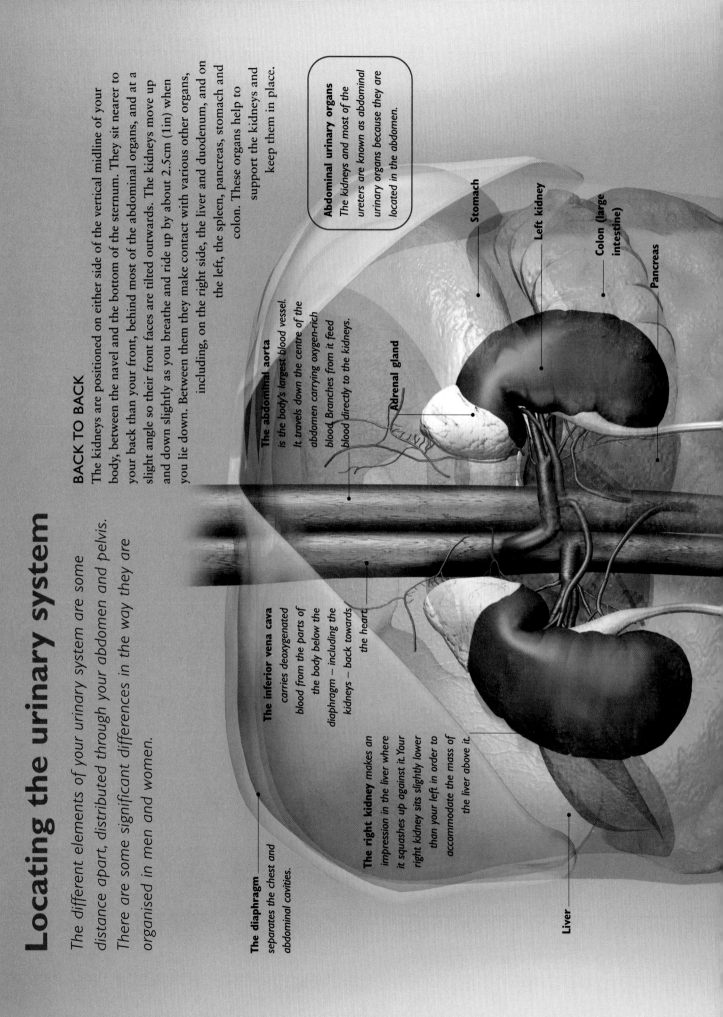

Abdominal urinary organs
The kidneys and most of the ureters are known as abdominal urinary organs because they are located in the abdomen.

Stomach

Left kidney

Colon (large intestine)

Pancreas

Adrenal gland

Liver

Prostate gland

MALE

The ureters pass down the back of the abdomen to the bladder.

Ureter

FEMALE

Bladder

Urethra

HOW MALE AND FEMALE URINARY SYSTEMS DIFFER

One of the main differences is the position of the bladder. In women it lies below the uterus and in front of the vagina, while in men it sits much higher, between the pubic bone and the rectum. The urethra in women is short and leads directly from the bladder down to an opening just in front of the vagina. In men, the urethra is much longer as it must pass through the centre of the prostate gland and then along the penis, to discharge via a narrow slit in the end of the penis.

The peritoneum
is a membranous bag that encloses the visceral organs such as the stomach, liver and intestines. The kidneys and ureters lie behind the peritoneum. Where they press against organs that move or change shape, such as the stomach, the peritoneum lubricates the contact so that there is no friction.

Pelvic urinary organs
The bladder and urethra are known as pelvic urinary organs because they are located in the pelvis.

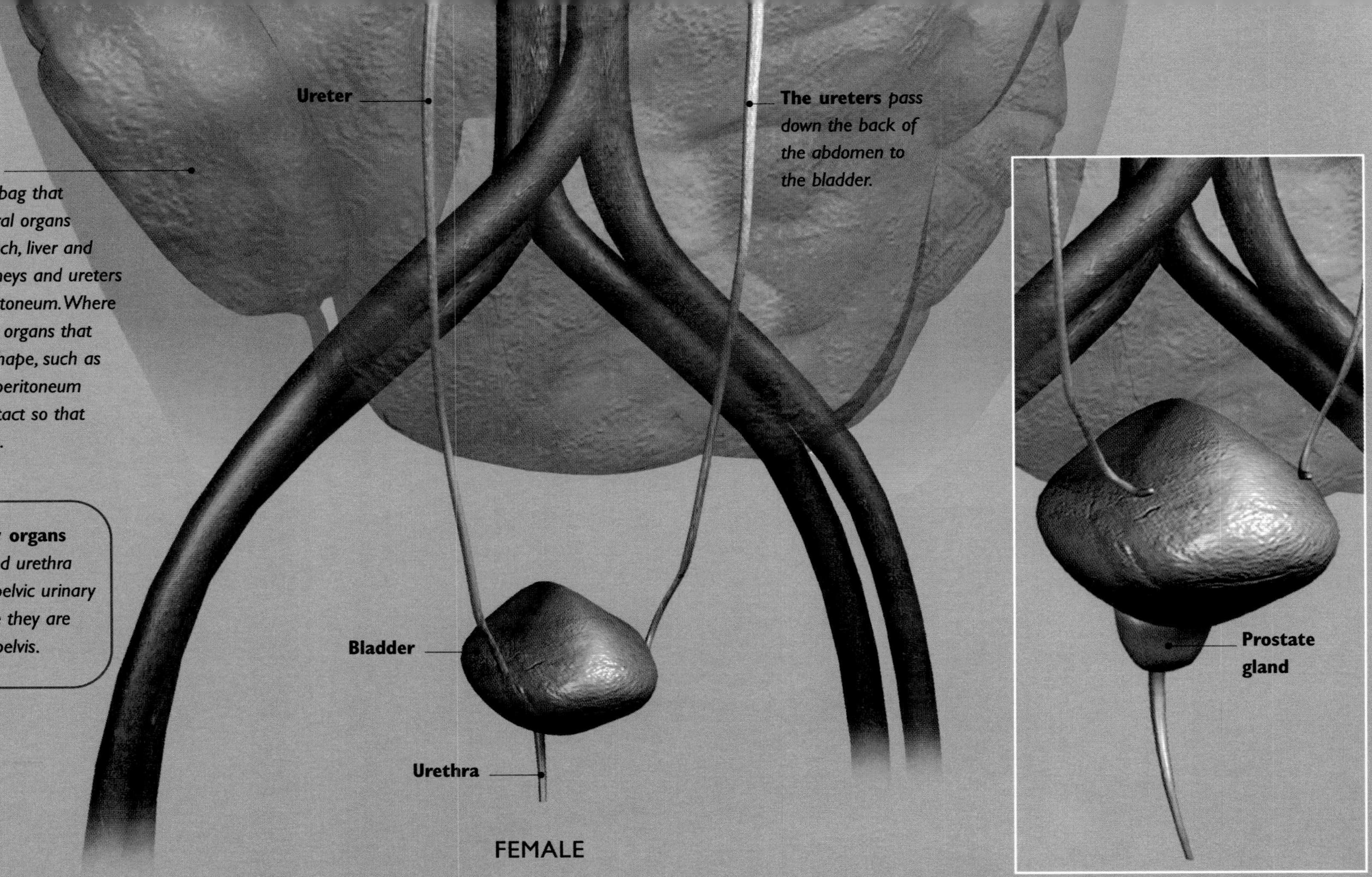

Point of view
This illustration shows the kidneys as if you were looking at them from the front, so the right kidney is shown on the left and vice versa. For greater clarity, the kidneys have been pulled forwards from their usual position in the abdominal cavity. In reality, they sit outside the peritoneum and behind the abdominal organs – such as the stomach, liver and intestines – that the peritoneum encloses.

The kidneys

The most vital parts of the urinary system are the kidneys. For protection, these delicate organs are carefully packed in protective tissue and sealed in the biological equivalent of shrink-wrapping.

Your kidneys process 600 times their own weight of fluid every day.

RIGHT KIDNEY

KIDNEY BEANS

Your kidneys are brownish-red bean-shaped organs, about 10cm (4in) long, 6cm (2¼in) wide and 3cm (1¼in) thick, and weighing about 150g (5¼oz) in men and slightly less – about 135g (4¾oz) – in women. They get their colour from the large number of blood vessels they contain. The inner edge of each kidney is concave, with a marked indentation in the middle: this is the hilum.

Functioning kidneys are essential to life, but a single kidney provides enough blood-processing capacity to keep the body in good health. The kidneys are not as well protected against injury as the heart and liver, and it seems likely that we have evolved two kidneys to safeguard against the loss of one due to an accident.

IN THE FLESH

Despite their distinctive appearance, the kidneys are actually quite hard to spot 'in the flesh' (during surgery, for instance), because each of them is wrapped up as carefully as a piece of fine bone china. The outermost layer of packaging is the renal capsule. There then follows another membrane, the renal fascia, which encloses a third layer – a layer of perirenal fat. The renal fascia and the perirenal (meaning 'enclosing the kidney') fat fuse with fascia (connective tissue) and fat that covers other tissues on the same region, including a band of fatty tissue that stretches all the way across the body to the other kidney.

The three layers provide plenty of protection while also keeping the kidneys firmly in place and immobilised. This is important because kidney function depends on the free flow of liquids through a variety of vessels and tubes, which must not get twisted or tangled.

The inner capsule of the kidney lies beneath the perirenal fat

The layer of perirenal fat that lies underneath the renal fascia is a mass of soft, cushioning, fatty tissue that helps to cushion and protect the kidney.

The renal fascia is a fibrous membrane of connective tissue that lies between the outer renal capsule and the layer of perirenal fat. The renal fascia is linked to the inner capsule by bridges of fibre that pass through the layer of fat.

The renal capsule is a tough, fibrous, outer membrane that encloses the renal fascia. It is bound to the renal fascia by fibrous bands called trabeculae.

The renal artery carries oxygenated blood from the abdominal aorta to the kidney.

LEFT KIDNEY

Adrenal gland

The adrenal glands are small endocrine (hormone-secreting) organs that sit atop the kidneys and even share some of their blood supply. They produce many important hormones, affect kidney function and interact with hormones produced by the kidney itself.

The hilum or 'root of the kidney' is where the major blood vessels and the ureter enter the interior of the kidney.

The renal vein takes deoxygenated blood from the kidney to the inferior vena cava and the heart.

Major calyx

The renal pelvis is an expansion of the ureter after it has entered the kidney. The renal pelvis subdivides into two or three major calyces.

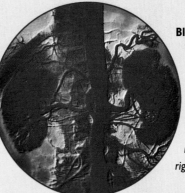

Blood rich
This arteriograph shows the abundant blood supply to the kidneys in red. The abdominal aorta runs down between the two kidneys and supplies each with oxygenated blood via the renal arteries which branch left and right directly from the aorta.

The ureter travels from the kidney to the bladder.

The internal structure of the kidney

The plain exterior of the kidney shields a fantastically intricate internal structure of pyramids, columns, funnels and rays, in which each element is minutely adapted to the organ's complex and continuous filtration process.

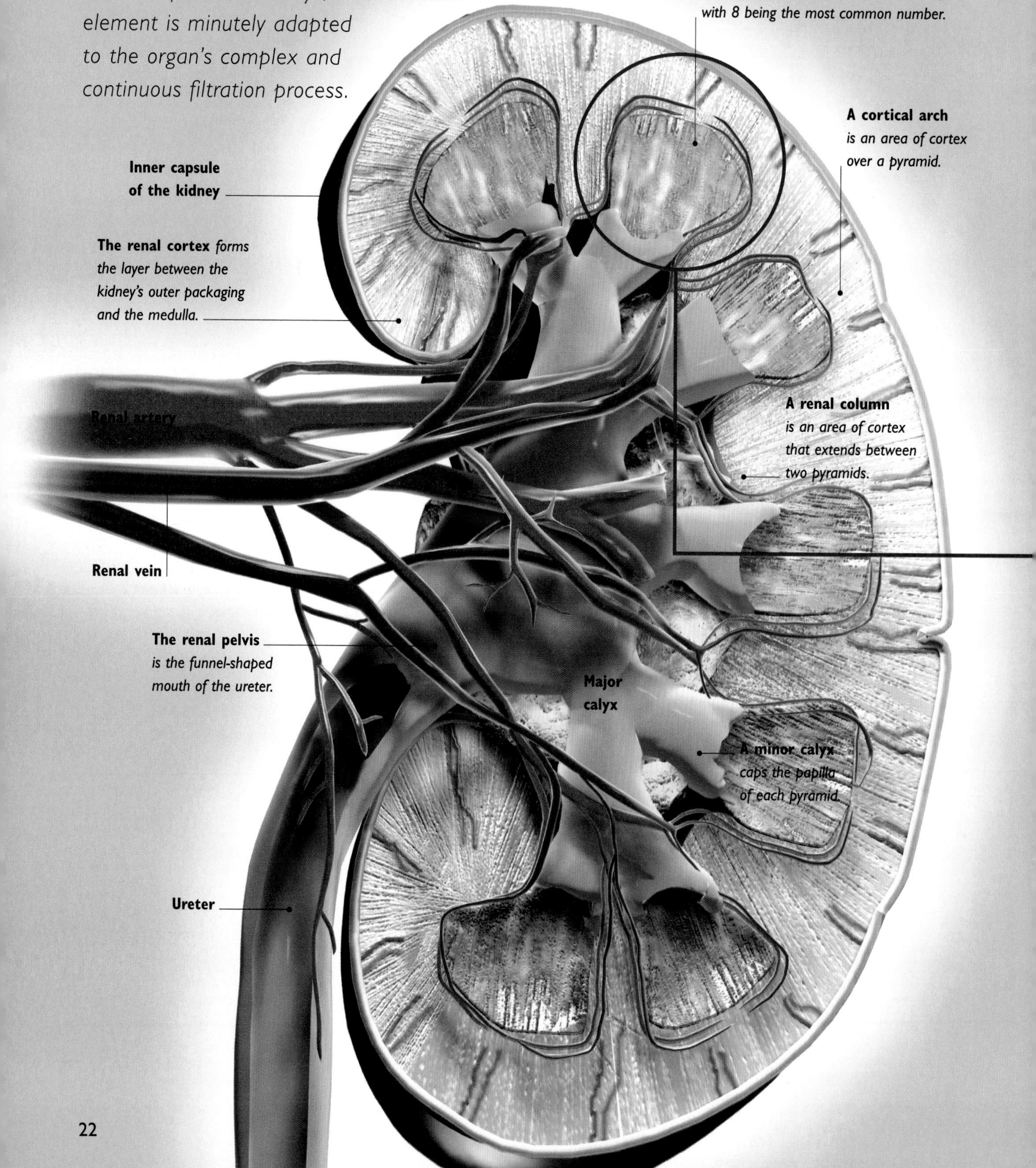

Each pyramid *forms a section within the medulla of the kidney. There are generally between 5 and 11 pyramids in a kidney, with 8 being the most common number.*

A cortical arch *is an area of cortex over a pyramid.*

Inner capsule of the kidney

The renal cortex *forms the layer between the kidney's outer packaging and the medulla.*

A renal column *is an area of cortex that extends between two pyramids.*

Renal artery

Renal vein

The renal pelvis *is the funnel-shaped mouth of the ureter.*

Major calyx

A minor calyx *caps the papilla of each pyramid.*

Ureter

THE PYRAMIDS

The main structural elements of the kidney are visible with the naked eye. A faintly stripy outer layer – the renal cortex – surrounds an inner layer known as the medulla, which is made up of pyramids. These are cones of tissue marked by grooves that converge towards the centre of the kidney. Between each pyramid, the cortex extends inwards in structures known as renal columns.

MILKING MACHINE

Each pyramid and the cortical arch above it make up a renal lobe, and the tip of each pyramid, the papilla, projects into a funnel-shaped piece of tissue called a minor calyx. The renal lobe produces urine which drains towards the papilla, where it drips out of tiny holes into the minor calyx. The word 'calyx' comes from the Latin for 'cup', and each minor calyx fits neatly over a papilla, rather like the cup of a milking machine on a cow's udder. Typically, a kidney has eight pyramids and therefore eight minor calyces. Two or more minor calyces feed into a major calyx, which decants in turn into the renal pelvis of the kidney (in an area known as the sinus) and then into the ureter.

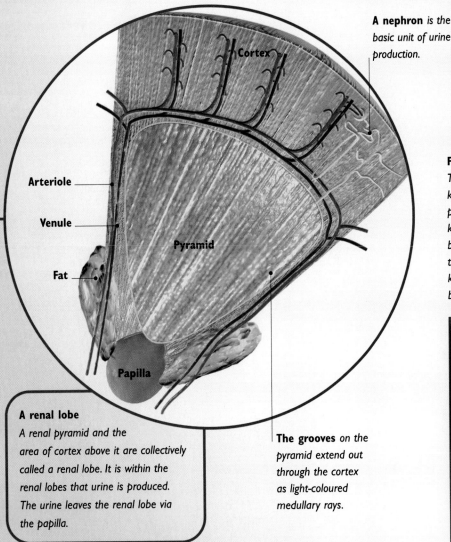

A nephron *is the basic unit of urine production.*

Cortex

Arteriole

Venule

Pyramid

Fat

Papilla

A renal lobe
A renal pyramid and the area of cortex above it are collectively called a renal lobe. It is within the renal lobes that urine is produced. The urine leaves the renal lobe via the papilla.

The grooves *on the pyramid extend out through the cortex as light-coloured medullary rays.*

From calyces to bladder
This coloured X-ray of the urinary tract – known as a urogram – clearly traces the path urine takes from the calyces within the kidneys to the bladder. Urograms are made by injecting an X-ray-opaque substance into the blood and then taking an X-ray after the kidneys have filtered the substance out of the blood and into the urinary system.

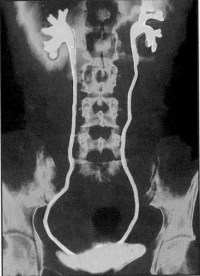

The nephron – an overview

The nephron is the basic structural and functional unit of the kidney. In each of your kidneys, these tiny units are busy round the clock, manufacturing urine and controlling the composition of your blood.

The average kidney contains some 1.25 million nephrons.

WHERE IT ALL HAPPENS

A nephron is essentially a long tube, with associated blood vessels; most nephrons are largely contained within the renal cortex and have loops of Henle that descend only a little way into the medulla, but some begin lower and extend deep into the medulla. At the top of the nephron is a structure called the renal corpuscle made up of the glomerulus and the Bowman's capsule. The renal tubule starts here, and almost immediately goes into a series of bends known as the proximal convoluted tubule (the PCT). The PCT leads to a length of tubule called the loop of Henle, which heads downwards and then turns back on itself until it ends in the twists and turns of the distal convoluted tubule (the DCT). Finally the DCT leads into what is known as the 'collecting system' – a series of tubules that collect urine and transport it to the tip of a renal pyramid.

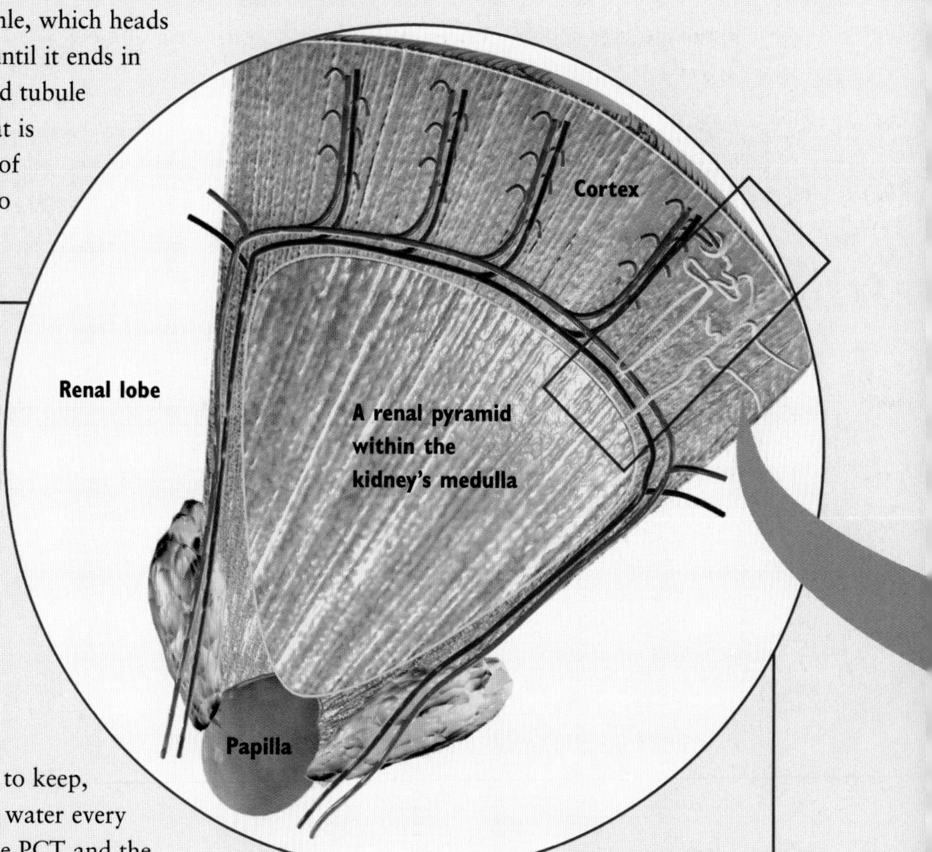

Cortex

Renal lobe

A renal pyramid within the kidney's medulla

Papilla

THE THREE STAGES OF URINE PRODUCTION

1 Filtration Urine starts off as 'filtrate' – essentially blood plasma (the nutrient-filled liquid in which red blood cells float) with the larger molecules filtered out. Filtration takes place in the glomeruli, which generate around 7 litres of filtrate every hour.

2 Reabsorption The filtrate is full of nutrients and ions that your body needs to keep, and you cannot afford to lose 7 litres of water every hour either. As filtrate passes through the PCT and the loop of Henle, most of the nutrients, ions and water are reabsorbed through the walls of the tubule into the bloodstream. Reabsorption also takes place in the DCT and the collecting tubules, but to a lesser degree. The amount of water and ions reabsorbed determines the make-up of your blood, its volume and pressure, and the amount and concentration of your urine.

3 Secretion As the filtrate passes through the DCT, substances are added to it. These include waste substances for excretion, drugs such as penicillin that your body wants to expel from the bloodstream, and a few ions to fine-tune the make up of your urine (and therefore the blood that is left behind).

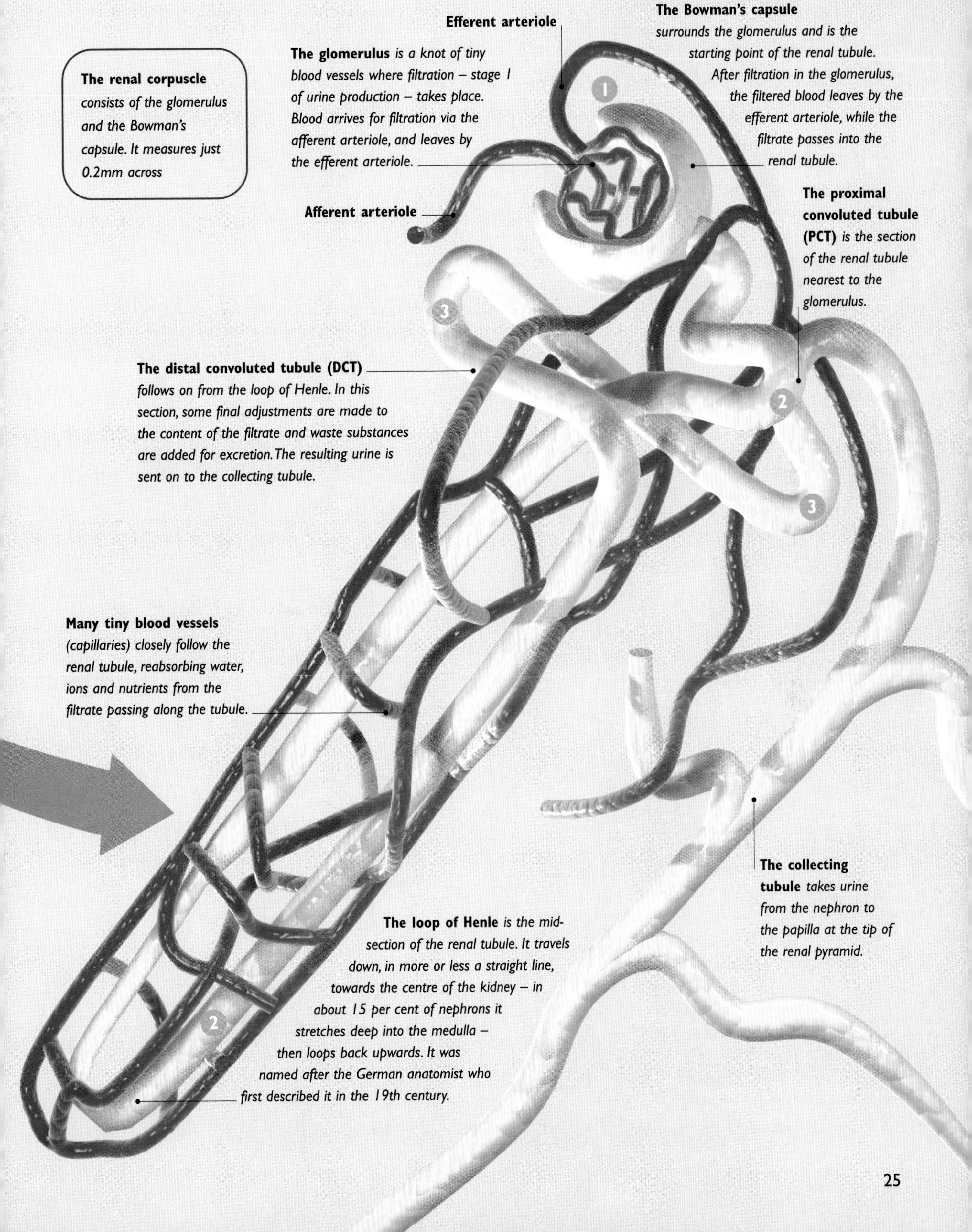

Efferent arteriole

The glomerulus *is a knot of tiny blood vessels where filtration – stage 1 of urine production – takes place. Blood arrives for filtration via the afferent arteriole, and leaves by the efferent arteriole.*

The Bowman's capsule *surrounds the glomerulus and is the starting point of the renal tubule. After filtration in the glomerulus, the filtered blood leaves by the efferent arteriole, while the filtrate passes into the renal tubule.*

The renal corpuscle *consists of the glomerulus and the Bowman's capsule. It measures just 0.2mm across*

Afferent arteriole

The proximal convoluted tubule (PCT) *is the section of the renal tubule nearest to the glomerulus.*

The distal convoluted tubule (DCT) *follows on from the loop of Henle. In this section, some final adjustments are made to the content of the filtrate and waste substances are added for excretion. The resulting urine is sent on to the collecting tubule.*

Many tiny blood vessels *(capillaries) closely follow the renal tubule, reabsorbing water, ions and nutrients from the filtrate passing along the tubule.*

The loop of Henle *is the mid-section of the renal tubule. It travels down, in more or less a straight line, towards the centre of the kidney – in about 15 per cent of nephrons it stretches deep into the medulla – then loops back upwards. It was named after the German anatomist who first described it in the 19th century.*

The collecting tubule *takes urine from the nephron to the papilla at the tip of the renal pyramid.*

25

The glomerulus

Inside the glomerulus, layers of cells build up around tiny blood vessels to make a finely tuned filter. This sieves all but the minutest molecules from the blood, turning it into the raw material for urine manufacture.

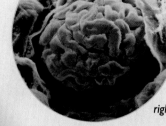

A glomerulus
A scanning electron micrograph (SEM) shows a glomerulus, with part of the Bowman's capsule visible as a white-brown membrane to the right of the glomerulus.

THE ALL-IMPORTANT FILTER

The tiny glomerulus sits inside the goblet-like Bowman's capsule at the blind end of the renal tubule. Blood arrives via the afferent arteriole, which enters the capsule through an opening called the vascular pole. The arteriole immediately splits into about 50 capillaries; these twine and knot around each other to form the glomerulus. The capillaries then join up again to form the efferent arteriole, which leaves via the vascular pole.

Fluid filters through the walls of the glomerulus and the inner walls of the capsule into its hollow interior – the capsular space – and then drains out of the 'stem' of the goblet into the proximal convoluted tubule.

The vascular pole
is where the arterioles leave and enter the Bowman's capsule.

The efferent arteriole
through which blood leaves the glomerulus.

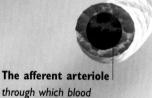

The afferent arteriole
through which blood enters the glomerulus.

Capillary

Capsular space

The Bowman's capsule *encloses the glomerulus. The outer walls of this hollow capsule make up the outer 'shell' of the corpuscle. The inner walls are made up of podocytes.*

Under pressure

The afferent arteriole is slightly wider than the efferent, so blood is delivered slightly faster than it can leave. This generates high blood pressure in the glomerulus, forcing the blood plasma through the glomerular filter. The walls of the afferent arteriole are ringed with muscle fibres that allow it to constrict and dilate. Constriction cuts pressure in the glomerulus because it reduces the blood flow, so less filtrate is produced; dilation has the opposite effect. This is one way the body controls how much urine is produced.

Flat, scale-like cells
form an inner lining to the wall of the Bowman's capsule.

Podocytes *are cells that bind to the walls of the glomerular capillaries and Bowman's capsule. They consist of a main cell body and many finger-like projections called pedicels or foot processes clearly seen in this SEM (right).*

Proximal convoluted tubule (PCT)

Cross-section through a capillary within a glomerulus

As blood flows down the capillary, water, ions and small molecules filter through the capillary walls into the capsular space. Blood remaining within the capillary continues down the network of capillaries surrounding the renal tubule and eventually enters a vein.

1 The fenestrae – *openings that perforate the capillary wall – are large enough to allow blood plasma through but not red blood cells.*

2 The glomerular basement membrane (GBM) *filters the blood plasma that has passed through the fenestrae.*

3 Podocytes *form the final barrier through which filtrate must pass before entering the Bowman's capsule.*

Filtrate escapes *into the hollow interior of the Bowman's capsule. At this stage of urine production the filtrate is rich in nutrients and other substances. It contains water, ions, waste products, glucose, fatty compounds, amino acids and vitamins.*

SUPER SIEVE

The filter that makes blood into filtrate is in several layers, each of which has progressively finer 'holes' – like a colander inside a sieve that is wrapped in muslin.

1 The 'colander' is the glomerular capillary. This has thousands of holes (called fenestrae, from the Latin for 'windows') which let blood plasma pass fairly freely, but are tiny enough to keep red blood cells inside.

2 The 'sieve' is the glomerular basement membrane (GBM). Basement membranes are found throughout the body, wherever a thin layer of cells acts as a barrier or wall of some sort. They act like a layer of biological 'mortar', holding cells together. The GBM is made up of the basement membrane of both the cells of the capillary wall and of the podocytes, and is unusually thick. Fluids and small and medium-sized molecules can pass through it, but it prevents the passage of the larger plasma proteins.

3 The final layer – the 'muslin' – is formed by the foot processes of the podocytes. These interlace, leaving tiny gaps called slit pores between them. The pores are covered in a clear, dense layer called the diaphragm, made up of two rows of interlocking filaments, a bit like a zip. Only water, small molecules and ions can pass through this layer.

Red blood cells *continue to flow down a capillary within the glomerulus.*

The renal tubule

The twists and turns of the renal tubule represent an intriguing puzzle. How do its coils and convolutions relate to its function of reclaiming vital substances before they are lost in the urine?

RECLAIMING NUTRIENTS FROM FILTRATE

Filtrate drains out of the Bowman's capsule into the proximal convoluted tubule (PCT) – the first section of the renal tubule. The walls of the PCT are made of cells packed with mitochondria – tiny biological engines that provide the energy to transport ions, organic nutrients and any plasma proteins that got through the glomerular filter out of the tubule and into the surrounding space, where they can be picked up by tiny blood vessels.

By moving these substances through the tubule wall, the PCT greatly increases the concentration of fluid outside the tubule. This attracts water from filtrate in the tubule, so water too passes through the wall to be reclaimed by the blood. Over 60 per cent of ions and water in the original filtrate are reclaimed in the PCT.

SALT SOLUTION

The PCT is followed by the loop of Henle, where reabsorption of filtrate into the blood continues. The ascending limb pumps salt ions out of the filtrate into the interstitial fluid outside the tubule. This fluid becomes very concentrated and draws more water from filtrate passing through the thin permeable sections of the loop. An additional 25 per cent of the water from the filtrate is reclaimed, as well as about 30 per cent of the ions and any remaining organic nutrients.

By the time the filtrate reaches the distal convoluted tubule (DCT) it contains little more than water, organic waste and a few ions. The DCT reabsorbs more salt ions and secretes substances into the filtrate, including waste matter and excess minerals that need to be removed from the blood. The DCT empties its load into a collecting tubule.

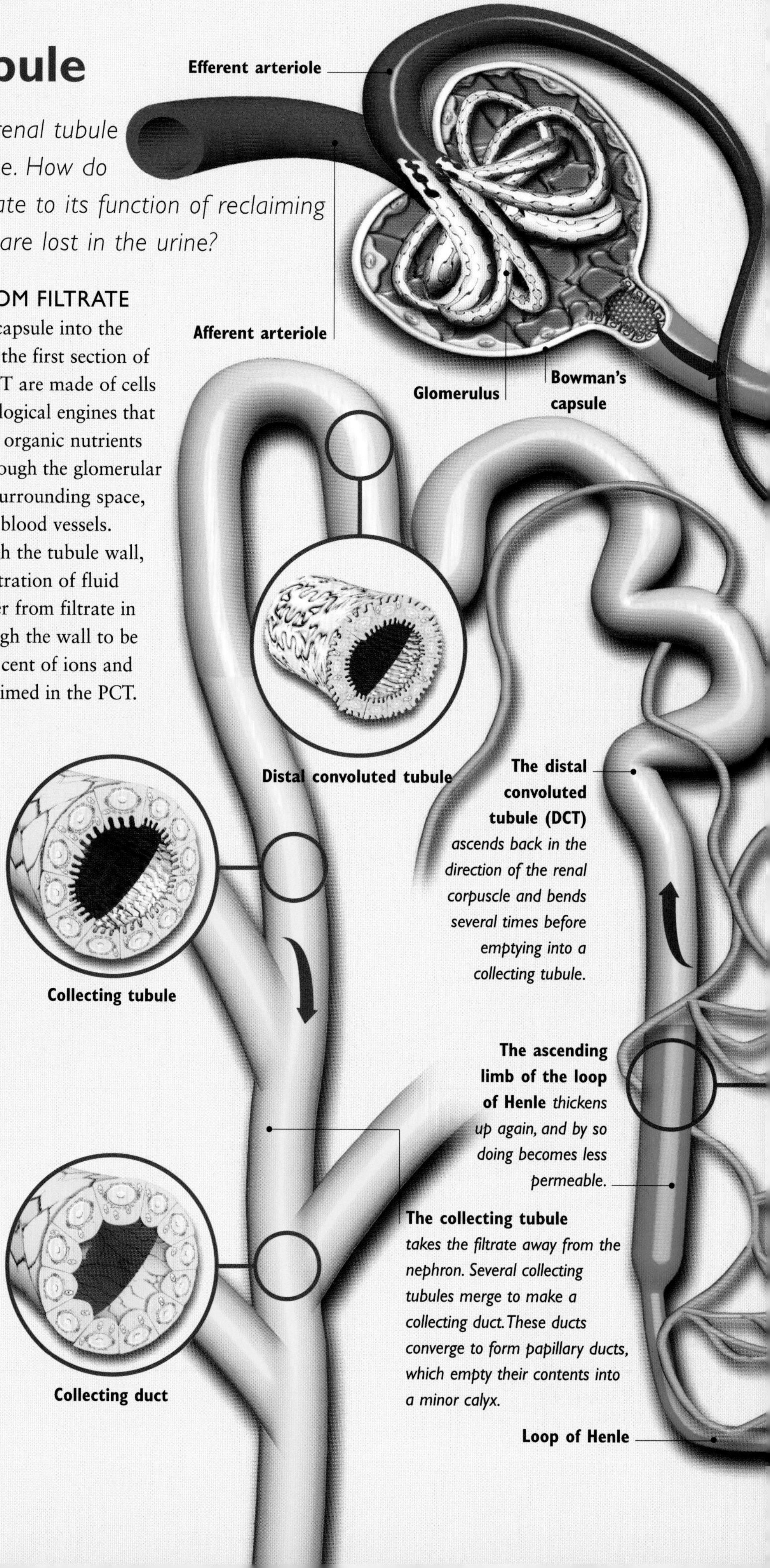

Efferent arteriole

Afferent arteriole

Glomerulus

Bowman's capsule

Distal convoluted tubule

Collecting tubule

Collecting duct

The distal convoluted tubule (DCT) *ascends back in the direction of the renal corpuscle and bends several times before emptying into a collecting tubule.*

The ascending limb of the loop of Henle *thickens up again, and by so doing becomes less permeable.*

The collecting tubule *takes the filtrate away from the nephron. Several collecting tubules merge to make a collecting duct. These ducts converge to form papillary ducts, which empty their contents into a minor calyx.*

Loop of Henle

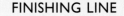

The proximal convoluted
tubule (PCT) *takes the
filtrate from the glomerulus
to the loop of Henle.*

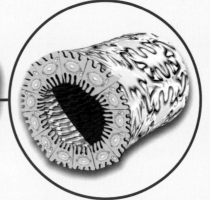

The vasa recta *is a network
of blood vessels that follows
the route of a renal tubule.
It absorbs water and
dissolved substances
reclaimed from the filtrate
and carries them back into
the circulation.*

Proximal convoluted tubule
*The PCT's thick walls are topped
with a forest of tiny hairs
called microvilli. These create a
huge surface area over which
the PCT can absorb water and
nutrients from the filtrate as it
passes along the tubule.*

FINISHING LINE

As each collecting tubule passes down through the medulla, it travels through the zone of highly concentrated fluid created by the loop of Henle. This fluid tends to draw water out of the filtrate, but the actual amount of water that is reabsorbed is determined by the permeability of the walls of the collecting tubule, which can be altered, allowing final adjustments to be made to the concentration of the filtrate. The degree of permeability is determined by levels of anti-diuretic hormone (ADH). High levels of this hormone make the collecting tubule more permeable, so that more water is reabsorbed – up to 95 per cent of the water content of the original filtrate can be reclaimed.

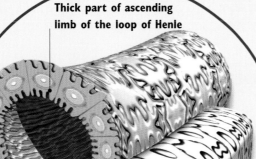

Thick part of ascending
limb of the loop of Henle

Capillaries belonging
to the vasa recta

The descending limb
of the loop of Henle
*becomes thinner and
highly permeable to water.*

Key
Afferent arteriole *Where blood enters the glomerulus.*
Efferent arteriole *The blood vessel that takes blood from the glomerulus to the vasa recta.*
Vasa recta *The network of small blood vessels – capillaries – that follows the course of the renal tubule.*
PCT *The proximal convoluted tubule of the nephron – the first part of the renal tubule.*
Loop of Henle *The mid-section of the renal tubule.*
DCT *The distal convoluted tubule – following on from the Loop of Henle.*
Collecting tubule *The tube that takes the filtrate from the nephron towards the renal pelvis of the kidney.*

A journey through the kidney

*A typical red blood cell travels through your kidneys 360 times
a day. Here you can follow one leg of this epic journey through
the kidney's complex web of arterioles, capillaries and venules.*

CRIMSON TIDE
Your kidneys receive 1.2 litres (about 2 pints) of blood every minute – about a quarter of the total output
of your heart. To deliver this enormous volume of blood your kidneys are well supplied with blood
vessels. The main supply comes from the renal artery, which splits off directly from the aorta. (In fact, just
under a third of people have an accessory renal artery – an extra artery supplying blood to the kidneys.)

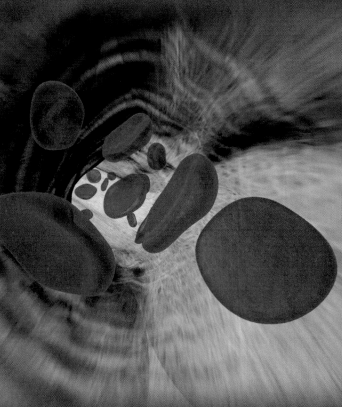

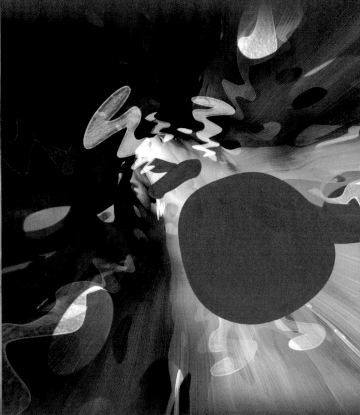

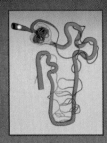

Travelling towards a nephron
Having left the renal artery to travel
down a wide segmental artery, the
red blood cell finds itself turning
down a side-branch and blasting
along an interlobar artery between
two pyramids in the medulla. Up
ahead the artery branches into the two arcuate arteries,
which carry blood along the border between the medulla
and cortex and deliver it to smaller arteries, which in turn
supply the afferent arterioles that feed the glomeruli.

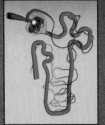

Into the glomerulus
Slowing down, the red blood cell
twists and turns as it is squeezed
through the knot of glomerular
capillaries. The pressure in the
glomerulus is tremendous, but the red
blood cell is too big to be forced
through one of the holes in the wall. The plasma around
it and smaller molecules such as glucose are draining out,
however. Any moment now the blood cell will be out of
the glomerulus and in the efferent arteriole.

The entire blood supply of your body passes through the kidneys roughly once every 4 minutes.

Rollercoaster ride
These computer-generated images are inspired by the journey a red blood cell travels as it passes through a kidney.

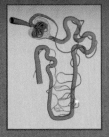

Going down the vasa recta

The efferent arteriole led into a bed of capillaries wrapped around the PCT (proximate convoluted tubule). Here, much of the fluid and nutrients extracted in the glomerulus rejoined the red blood cell. Now the blood cell is falling down a vessel that is part of the vasa recta – the network of capillaries around the loop of Henle. Nearby is a blood vessel going the other way – the ascending limb of the vasa recta – and our cell will soon be travelling up it.

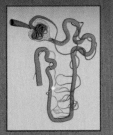

Ion exchange

The ascending vasa recta is full of salt ions, picked up from the salty fluid in the medulla. These ions need to remain in the medulla. The two blood vessels are parallel so ions from the ascending limb can pass into the descending limb, and be carried down into the medulla. It's a contraflow system, called the counter-current exchange system. From the vasa recta, our blood cell passes along a venule and a series of larger veins until it returns to the main circulation.

The adrenal glands

Apart from maintaining blood composition and making urine, the kidneys are also important sites of hormone production. Hormones are made both within the kidneys themselves and by the adrenal glands that sit on top of them.

YELLOW CAP

Sitting on top of each of your kidneys is a pyramid-shaped mass of yellow tissue called the adrenal gland. One of the most important and prolific glands in your body, the adrenal gland produces hormones that play a role in everything from sex and fighting to arthritis and blood pressure. Although part of the endocrine system rather than the urinary system, the adrenal glands interact with and affect kidney function.

Hormone production

Each adrenal gland has two main parts: an inner medulla and an outer cortex. The cortex uses the lipids it stores to manufacture 'steroid' hormones, including sex hormones and anti-inflammatory corticosteroids. One such hormone is aldosterone, an anti-diuretic hormone that signals the kidneys to reabsorb sodium ions and water and thus produce less urine.

The medulla itself produces mainly adrenaline. As part of the 'fight-or-flight' response, this potent hormone triggers the mobilisation of energy reserves in the body and generally helps it gear up for action.

A tough, fibrous capsule *protects the adrenal glands and also binds them firmly to the kidney's own capsule.*

Adrenal gland

A branch of the suprarenal artery *carries blood into the adrenal gland.*

Outer renal capsule of the kidney

Blood supply to the adrenal glands
The adrenal glands need to deliver their product to the rest of the body as quickly as possible. Accordingly they are well supplied with blood, from the suprarenal arteries and branches of other arteries including the renal artery.

KIDNEY-GROWN HORMONES

The kidney's endocrine functions are performed by the juxtaglomerular apparatus (JGA), a conglomeration of cells next to each glomerulus. The JGA monitors blood pressure and volume, making and secreting renin and erythropoietin into the bloodstream if a drop is detected. The enzyme renin boosts levels of the hormone angiotensin by converting it from an inactive to an active form. Angiotensin triggers the release of aldosterone by the adrenal glands, which leads to increased salt and water re-uptake and higher blood pressure and volume. Erythropoietin boosts red blood cell production and therefore blood volume.

Negative feedback loop

The interaction between the adrenal gland and the JGA is an example of a negative feedback loop – a control mechanism that prevents hormonal responses from getting out of control. In this case aldosterone reduces the stimulus for its own production by increasing blood pressure. This causes the JGA to stop making renin, so that angiotensin levels fall and no longer trigger aldosterone production.

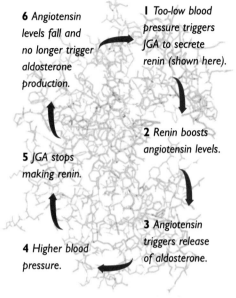

6 Angiotensin levels fall and no longer trigger aldosterone production.

1 Too-low blood pressure triggers JGA to secrete renin (shown here).

2 Renin boosts angiotensin levels.

5 JGA stops making renin.

3 Angiotensin triggers release of aldosterone.

4 Higher blood pressure.

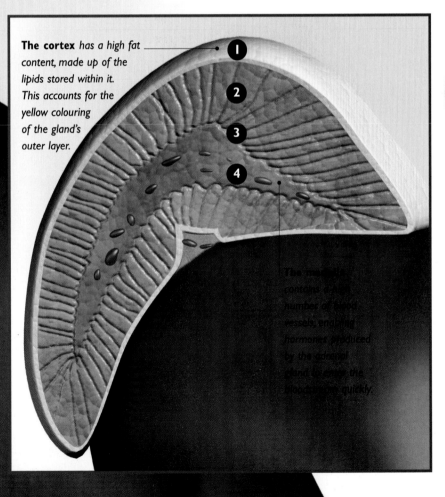

The cortex has a high fat content, made up of the lipids stored within it. This accounts for the yellow colouring of the gland's outer layer.

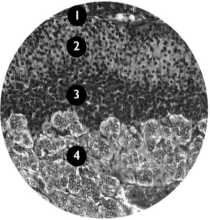

The cortex and medulla
The adrenal cortex has three layers, each of which produces different types of hormone:
1 The zona glomerulosa produces the hormone aldosterone.
2 The zona fasciculata produces glucocorticoids that help to regulate glucose metabolism in the body.
3 The zona reticulans produces androgens – male sex hormones – in both genders.

In the centre of the gland, surrounded by the cortex, is the medulla (labelled **4**). The medulla secretes the hormones adrenaline and noradrenaline. In all, the adrenal gland produces more than 30 different hormones.

The ureters and the bladder

The collection and storage elements of the urinary system are relatively simple but robust organs, designed to handle large and small volumes of urine with equal efficiency, and to ensure it flows in one direction only.

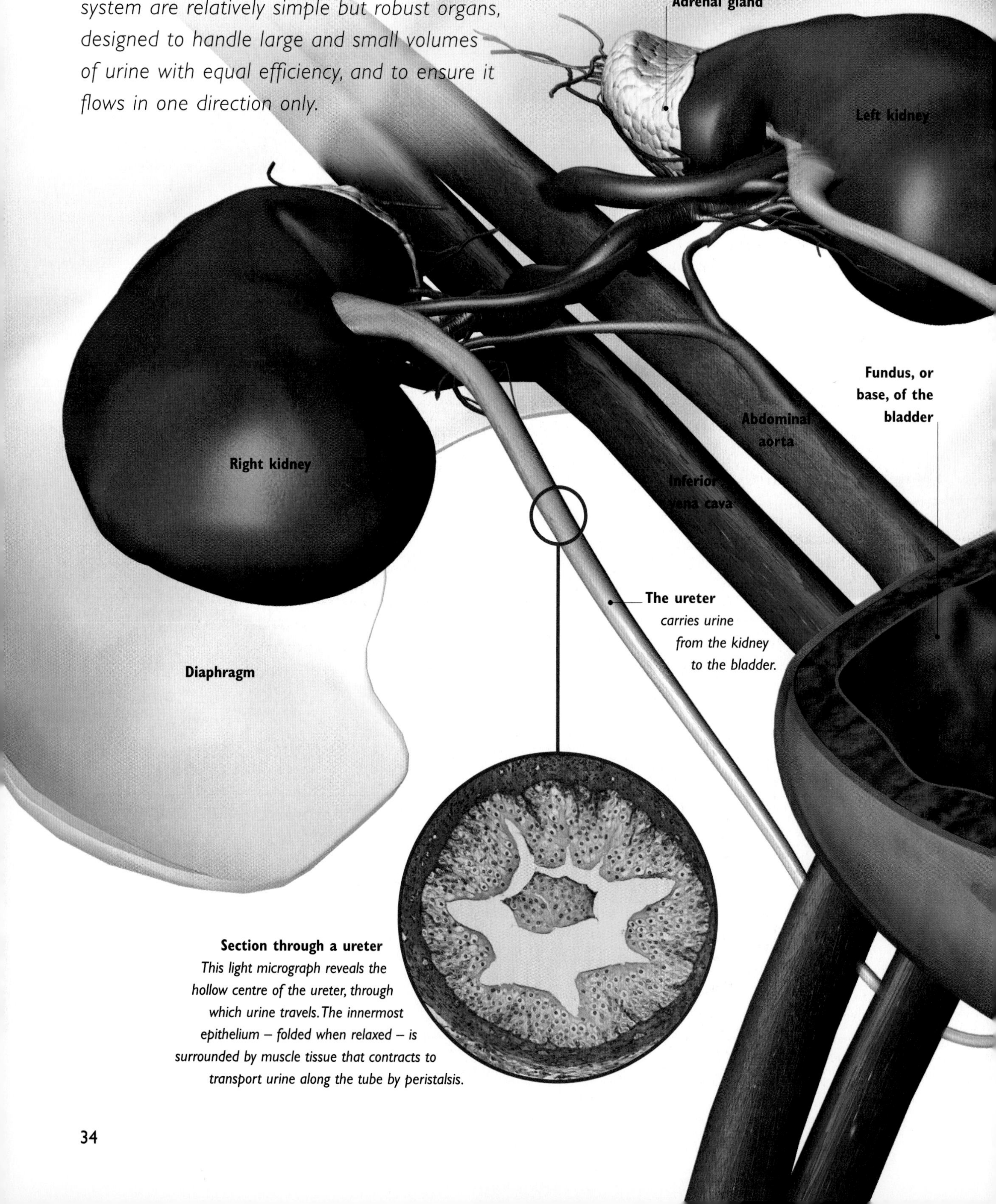

Adrenal gland

Left kidney

Right kidney

Fundus, or base, of the bladder

Abdominal aorta

Inferior vena cava

The ureter
carries urine from the kidney to the bladder.

Diaphragm

Section through a ureter
This light micrograph reveals the hollow centre of the ureter, through which urine travels. The innermost epithelium – folded when relaxed – is surrounded by muscle tissue that contracts to transport urine along the tube by peristalsis.

TAKING THE TUBE

Urine is transported from the kidneys to the bladder via a pair of 25–30cm (10–12in) long muscular tubes called the ureters. The ureters begin inside the kidneys, where the funnel-like calyces empty urine into the renal pelvis, which forms the entrance to the ureter. Waves of contraction begin in the muscular calyces and travel along the ureter, pushing urine towards the bladder. In a normal bladder, contractions occur every 20–30 seconds.

One way only

When the ureters reach the bladder, they pass through its wall at an angle, each ending in a slit-like opening designed to prevent urine flowing back up towards the kidney. As the bladder fills with urine and expands, the bladder walls stretch, causing the slit to squeeze more tightly shut and pressing on the ureter where it passes through the bladder wall, again helping to close it off.

IN THE BAG

Your bladder is a hollow, muscular bag that acts as an expandable temporary urine reservoir. When empty it sits in your lower pelvis, but as it fills it expands upwards and forwards. In a normal adult the bladder rarely holds more than 320ml (just over half a pint) of urine, with the urge to urinate coming at the 280ml mark. More than 500ml (a little less than one pint) causes pain and an intense urge to urinate immediately.

A layer of mucous membrane lines the inside of the bladder. It is arranged in folds, called rugae, so that the lining can expand as the bladder fills with urine.

The ureters enter the bladder about three-quarters of the way down the bladder wall. The two entrance slits are about 5cm (2in) apart when the bladder is full.

Small volumes of urine flow from the kidneys to the bladder roughly once every 25 seconds or so.

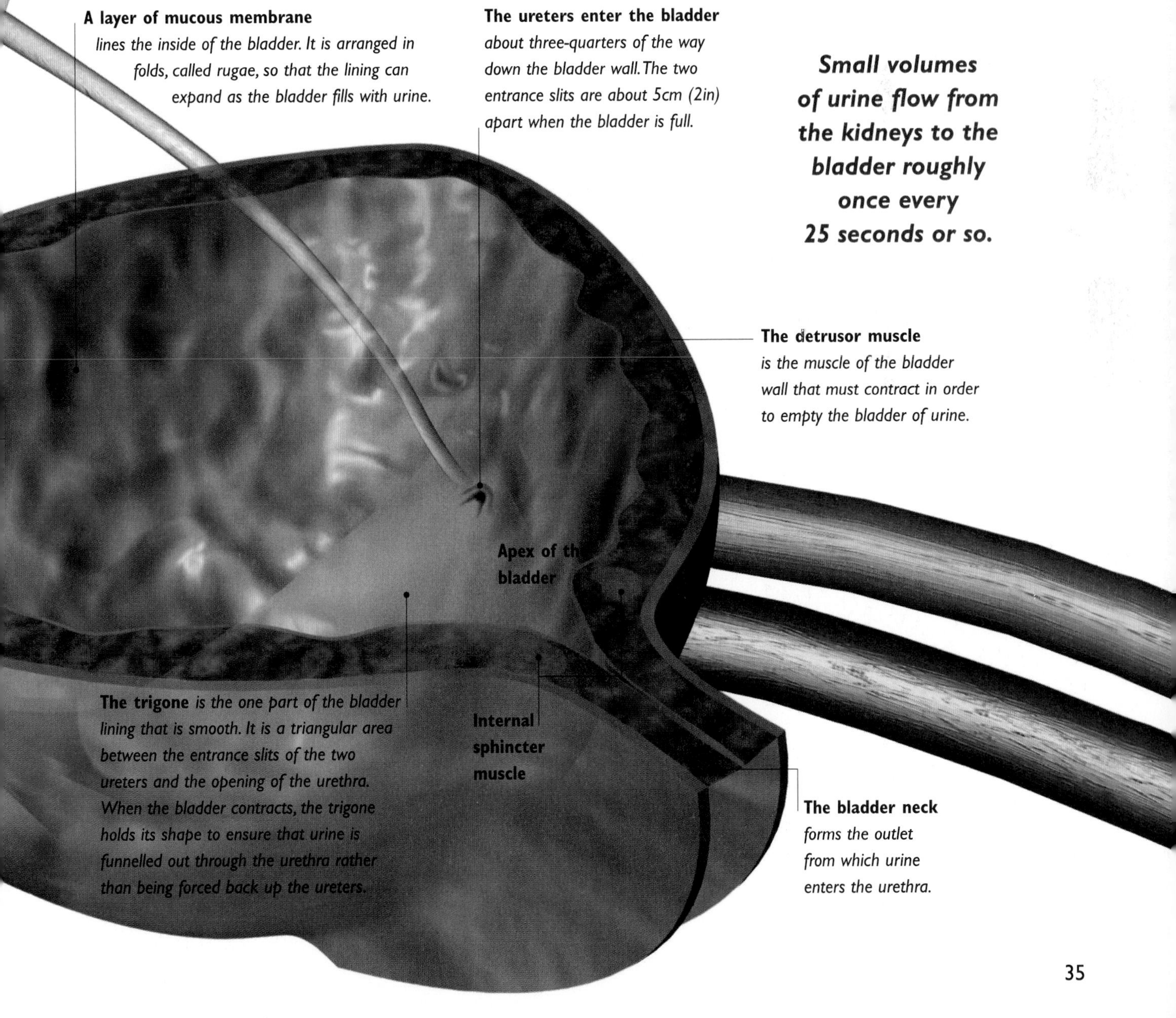

The detrusor muscle is the muscle of the bladder wall that must contract in order to empty the bladder of urine.

Apex of the bladder

The trigone is the one part of the bladder lining that is smooth. It is a triangular area between the entrance slits of the two ureters and the opening of the urethra. When the bladder contracts, the trigone holds its shape to ensure that urine is funnelled out through the urethra rather than being forced back up the ureters.

Internal sphincter muscle

The bladder neck forms the outlet from which urine enters the urethra.

The urethra and urination

The final stage in the journey of urine from kidney to toilet is along the urethra, a narrow tube that bears responsibility for providing continence – the ability to control when and where urine is released.

Urine gets its colour from a nitrogen-containing pigment called urochrome.

THE SHORT AND THE LONG

The urethra is a muscular tube that transports urine from the bladder neck to the external opening of the urinary system. It differs considerably between the sexes, not least in length: in men it is five times as long as it is in women. In men it also overlaps with the reproductive system.

In both men and women, there is a ring of muscle where the urethra passes through the pelvic floor muscles. This is the external urethral sphincter, which is under a person's conscious voluntary control.

KEEPING CONTROL

Continence depends on the pressure in the urethra being higher than the pressure in the bladder. As long as this is the case, urine will not flow out of the bladder. High urethral pressure is maintained mainly by the external sphincter, helped by elastic fibres in the neck of the bladder. Urination, or, as it is more commonly called in medical circles, micturition, involves reversing this state of affairs, first by decreasing pressure in the urethra and then by increasing the pressure in the bladder, using a combination of voluntary and involuntary mechanisms.

Men only

In men the urethra carries semen as well as urine. As the urethra passes through the prostate gland, the ejaculatory duct from the testes and the prostate itself feed into the urethra, bringing sperm and semen fluid. Just above the prostate, where the urethra exits the bladder, there is a build up of muscle fibres that forms an internal urethral sphincter, which is believed to help prevent the flow of semen the wrong way up the urethra.

Internal urethral sphincter muscle

Ureter

Rectum

Bladder

Pubic bone

The penile or spongiose urethra *is 15cm long, and has a diameter of 6mm when passing urine.*

The prostate gland *becomes enlarged with age and may obstruct the prostatic urethra and bladder neck, impairing urination.*

The prostatic urethra *is 3–4cm long.*

Pelvic floor muscles

The urethra in men
A man's urethra is 18–20cm (7–7.5in) long and it has different names along its length. The first section is called the 'prostatic' urethra because it passes through the prostate gland. The next section cuts through the pelvic floor muscles and is known as the 'membranous' urethra. The final section, the 'penile' or 'spongiose' urethra, is the longest part and ends in a small slit in the tip of the glans.

The membranous urethra *passes through the external urethral sphincter and pelvic floor muscles; it is just 1.8cm long.*

Testicle

Urethral opening

THE PROCESS OF URINATION

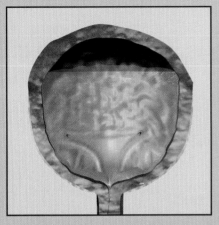 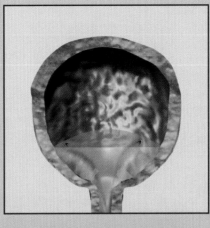 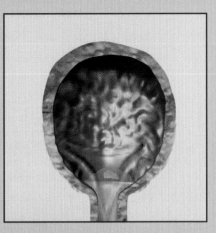

1 *When the bladder is full enough for urination to be desirable, stretch receptors in the bladder wall send signals to an area of the spinal cord called the micturition reflex centre (MRC). This alerts the brain, which produces a conscious urge to urinate but also blocks the MRC from going any further at this point.*

2 *Once the decision to urinate has been made, and the external sphincter muscle has been voluntarily relaxed, urination can begin. The brain stops inhibiting the MRC and amplifies the signals it transmits. The nervous impulses from the bladder stretch receptors now trigger the full micturition reflex.*

3 *The MRC orders the bladder's detrusor muscles to contract, forcing the urine out of the bladder, down the urethra and past the relaxed external sphincter to the outside of the body. As soon as the bladder has emptied the detrusor muscle relaxes and the external sphincter become tightly closed once more.*

Ureter

Uterus

Bladder

Rectum

Pubic
bone

Bladder neck

Urethra

Pelvic floor
muscles

**The external
sphincter**
*surrounds the
urethra as it passes
through the pelvic
floor muscles.*

The vestibule
*is the space into
which the urethra
and vagina open.
It is bounded by
the labia minora.*

The urethra in women
*A woman's urethra is only 4cm (1.5in)
long. It passes through the pelvic floor
muscles just in front of the vagina,
and opens onto the vestibule.*

Vaginal
opening

Urethral
opening

A day in the life of the urinary system

Your kidneys are hard at work all day manufacturing urine, and in the process maintaining the healthy composition of your blood. The urinary tract and bladder then take charge to arrange the transport, storage and safe disposal of the urine.

MIND CONTROL

Control of the urinary system involves a complex web of coordinated mechanisms, some conscious and some unconscious. Each mechanism is directed by a different system, yet they all work together to ensure the smooth running of the urinary system overall. Control systems of which you are quite unaware are constantly monitoring your blood, sending and receiving hormonal and nervous messages, monitoring feedback from each other, and alerting your conscious mind when you need to take appropriate actions, such as drinking or urinating.

07:00 Wake up call

Your buzzer wasn't set to go off for another 15 minutes when alarm signals of another kind rouse you from slumber. After more than 7 hours of solid sleep, the micturition reflex centre (MRC) in your spine says it's time to get up: alerted by signals from the stretch receptors in the bladder wall, working via the cortex of your brain, the MRC produces a strong urge to urinate. When you relieve yourself you notice that your urine is dark yellow – this is because, with no fluid coming in while you slept, your kidneys have retained as much water in the body as they can, producing a concentrated urine.

20:00 Added extras

Your takeaway pizza is deliciously tasty; one reason is that the dough and the toppings are laden with salt (sodium chloride) – far more than you'd normally use. Soon the concentration of sodium ions in your bloodstream is climbing beyond optimal limits; you need more water in your blood to help to dilute the salt. 'Osmoreceptor' cells in the hypothalamus detect the increased blood concentration and stimulate your pituitary gland to make antidiuretic hormone (ADH). ADH increases the permeability of the collecting tubules in your kidneys, so that they allow more water to be reabsorbed into the bloodstream. At the same time your nervous system signals the nephrons to retain more sodium inside the PCT and loop of Henle, so that more is excreted into the urine.

13:30 Lunch time at the gym

You take off at lunch time for a session at the local gym. As you work away on an exercise bike, your body temperature rises and your sweating mechanism comes into play to bring your temperature back to where it should be, at around 37°C. As well as helping you to cool down, sweating is another way in which water and waste products are expelled from the body, other than through the urinary system. It's time to drink some more water.

11:30 Thirsty work

Thanks to the coffee this is the second time you've been to the loo since you got to work. This means you've lost quite a lot of water, resulting in a small drop in blood volume. The drop is detected by the juxtaglomerular apparatus (JGA) next to each glomerulus, causing the granular cells of the JGA to release renin into your bloodstream. The renin activates angiotensin, which triggers the hypothalamus in your brain to create a sensation of thirst by reducing saliva production from the salivary glands. The resulting dry mouth and throat send you to the water cooler.

09:30 Morning coffee

A couple of cups of coffee have given you a caffeine boost, but caffeine is a diuretic, affecting your nephrons in several ways. Firstly it causes a slight increase in blood pressure, producing more filtrate in the glomeruli. Secondly it affects the tubules, causing them to reabsorb less water as the filtrate passes through. Soon your bladder is filling up fast – it won't be long before you have to go again.

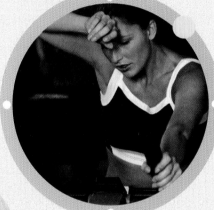

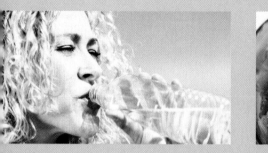 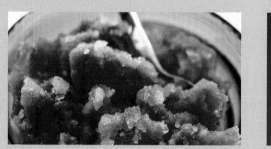 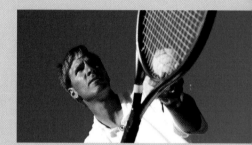

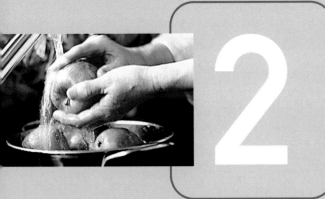

2

Healthy kidneys for life

KEEPING YOUR URINARY SYSTEM HEALTHY

For most people most of the time, the health of their urinary system is in their own hands: healthy habits through life's various stages, an awareness of potential hazards and an informed use of medications can go a long way to keeping the kidneys and urinary system in optimum health.

43 *Bladder problems are often quickly apparent, but keeping an eye on what's normal for you can alert you to potential problems early.*

47 *Pregnancy is a time of enormous change, when many factors impact on the urinary system – read what to expect at this exciting time.*

48 *Simple changes to bathroom habits can have an enormous impact on urinary health: learn what you can do to keep the system working well.*

52 *What you wear and how you launder clothes can mean the difference between good and poor health for your urinary system.*

54 *The world around us is generally safer than it has been for generations, but there are still hazards that can harm the kidneys.*

57 *As the kidneys are prime filters of toxins, any medication – prescribed, over-the-counter or herbal – might prove to be a threat to health.*

Knowing what's normal for you

A healthy urinary system requires little maintenance, but since symptoms of bladder and kidney problems can be painful, embarrassing and irritating, it is well worth being able to spot the early signs if something is wrong.

GET TO KNOW YOUR BODY

The first step in recognising possible problems is to know what is normal for you. By taking a little time to establish what is normal, you are more likely to realise quickly when something is wrong.

Some signs of urinary infection come on fast and are easy to spot: the painful urination associated with a urinary tract infection can quickly be assessed. Other symptoms are more insidious and can take weeks or even months to become apparent.

Frequency of bathroom trips

Most bladders hold between 300 and 600ml (½ to 1 pint) of urine. These amounts do vary from person to person, so don't worry if you are a little different. It is often a change in normal habits that may signal a problem: needing to urinate every hour, for example, when you have not been used to doing so.

It is important to know that many problems can be helped – or even cured – if they are spotted early.

TAKE CHARGE OF BLADDER HEALTH

Think about the following factors. If your answers suggest a problem with urine or bladder control, see your doctor.

On average, how often do you empty your bladder during the day?
The normal range is from six to eight times a day.

Do you wake up during the night to empty your bladder? If so, how often?
Once during the night is nothing to worry about, but more may indicate a problem and can be debilitating.

How much urine do you pass each time you visit the bathroom? Does it vary?
The urge to pass urine is not usually triggered until there is between 150 and 350ml – about a glassful.

Does your bladder feel empty after urination?
If the bladder has difficulty emptying and urine dribbles out rather than flowing freely this may indicate overflow incontinence. This could be caused by a blockage at the neck of the bladder or an enlarged prostate.

What does your urine normally look like?
Urine should be a pale straw colour, but if you become dehydrated then it becomes more concentrated and so a darker colour. It is normal for this to happen overnight, with morning urine being darker.

What does it smell like? Does it smell unusual?
A strong ammonia smell may indicate an infection.

Are there times of the day when you pass more urine? Does anything seem to make you pass more or less urine?
Tea, coffee, chocolate, sweeteners, cola, acidic or spicy foods, can all irritate the bladder and intensify any urinary tract symptoms.

How does drinking alcohol affect your pattern of urination?
Alcohol can affect bladder control, increase urination and aggravate incontinence problems.

Do you ever leak urine when you laugh, cough or sneeze?
This may indicate a weakening of the tissues supporting the bladder, causing stress incontinence.

Is passing urine ever painful?
Passing urine should not be painful. Pain may indicate an infection, or be caused by something pressing on the bladder, such as a cyst or stone.

Are you unable to control the urge to urinate, and leak urine? Do you wet the bed at night?
Such incontinence can be caused by a bladder or urinary tract infection, or may suggest a malfunction of nerves in the brain, spinal cord or surrounding the bladder.

Do you get urinary tract infections? How frequently? Does anything in particular seem to trigger a urinary infection?
For example exercise, medication, sex, anxiety or stress, excessive fluid intake or dehydration.

THE BENEFITS OF
URINARY HEALTH

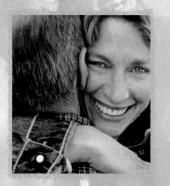

SATISFYING RELATIONSHIPS
A sexual relationship can be enjoyed without fear of pain or embarrassment.

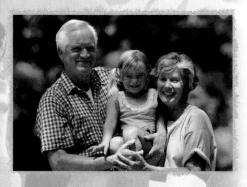

GOOD QUALITY SLEEP
Uninterrupted sleep helps give you the energy to meet your commitments.

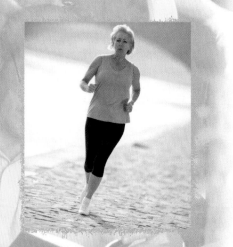

HEALTH-GIVING EXERCISE
Exercise and all its many health benefits – increased energy, weight control, improved sleep patterns etc. – can be pursued free from the worry of leakage or pain.

COMMON PROBLEMS

Among the most common problems affecting the urinary tract and kidneys are incontinence, urinary tract infections and kidney stones. While none of these are life threatening, they can cause pain or discomfort. More serious and potentially life-threatening – though with symptoms similar to a urinary tract infection – is bladder cancer.

Estimates suggest that as many as 50 per cent of women suffer from incontinence at some time in their lives.

A hyperactive bladder

Older people in particular may experience what is known as a hyperactive bladder. Someone with a hyperactive bladder has the urge to pass urine frequently, but is only able to pass small amounts of urine each time. This is because the bladder contracts involuntarily and too frequently, but not enough to empty the bladder completely. This condition can lead to urine overflowing and leaking involuntarily from the bladder. The only way to empty the bladder completely in such cases is by straining down – which may damage or weaken the bladder and urethra – or by emptying the bladder using a catheter.

Urinary tract infections (UTIs)

Urinary tract infections (UTIs) vary from mild inflammations of the urethra and bladder (cystitis) to more serious infections of the kidney, which may have travelled up the urinary tract to one or both kidneys.

UTIs are much more frequent in women than men. However, in older age groups, after the age of 60 or so, almost as many men suffer from infections as women.

The term cystitis covers a range of infections and irritations of the lower urinary tract. The most common cause of cystitis is bacteria from the anus which have travelled up the urethra and into the bladder. If the bladder is emptied fairly frequently, these bacteria can be prevented from settling and causing problems. If a person is unable to empty the bladder completely – for example, a man with an enlarged prostate – bacteria are not flushed out of the system and as a result can cause infection. People most prone to cystitis are:
- women and girls, because they have a shorter urethra than men and therefore bacteria have less distance to travel up the urethra before reaching the bladder;
- pregnant women;
- post-menopausal women;
- those who have a congenital problem in their urinary system;
- men with an enlarged prostate gland;
- people who have to empty their bladder by using a catheter.

Symptoms can include some or all of the following:
- a frequent desire to pass urine;
- a burning sensation or pain, when passing urine;
- cloudy and strong-smelling urine – some might describe it as ammonia-like or 'fishy-smelling';
- pain above the pubic bone, in the lower abdomen;
- a general feeling of fever or nausea, or flu-like symptoms;
- kidney pain.

Interstitial cystitis (IC)

Interstitial cystitis (IC) is also known as painful bladder syndrome or frequency-urgency-dysuria syndrome. This chronic disorder is often overlooked or misdiagnosed, especially in its early stages. Symptoms vary, but usually include:

• a decreased bladder capacity;
• an urgent and frequent need to empty the bladder, day and night;
• pain and tenderness in the bladder, pelvis and perineum;
• difficulty sitting or driving a car;
• sensitivity to acidic foods;
• pain on sexual intercourse.

The symptoms may be mistaken for those of an ordinary urinary tract infection, but they do not subside, even after repeated courses of antibiotics; in fact, they may even become more acute and debilitating. Approximately nine out of ten of all sufferers are women, mostly between the ages of 20 and 50. Patients with IC are 10–12 times more likely to report childhood bladder problems, and IC is often diagnosed only after all other urinary conditions which have similar symptoms have been ruled out.

The exact cause of IC is unknown. In the past it was thought to be of an emotional or psychological nature, because no evidence of bacteria was found in the urine. It is now accepted that interstitial cystitis is a very real disease, and research and treatment focus on the lining of the bladder. This lining usually protects the bladder from the toxic effects of urine. However, in 70 per cent of interstitial cystitis sufferers the lining of the bladder is found to be 'leaky', and it is thought that substances pass through the bladder wall to trigger the symptoms of IC.

Kidney stones

Stones formed in the kidneys are usually made of calcium, though some may be formed of oxalate, cystine or struvite – all by-products of the chemical and physical changes that take place within the body. People who experience pain from kidney stones tend to be between the ages of 20 and 50, with stones occurring more frequently in men than women.

Generally, kidney stones are small enough to move down the ureter, into the bladder and out of the body without becoming stuck along the way. This journey can sometimes be painful, however, with nausea and vomiting as well as pain on one side of the back and/or in the stomach or groin area. The pain should stop once the stones have been excreted with urine. If a stone gets stuck at some point along the urinary tract the pain will continue and a visit to the hospital for pain control and, if necessary, removal of the stone is usually in order.

Not all kidney stones cause pain: many pass along the urinary tract without incident because they are so small, while others do not move from the kidney at all.

Most kidney stones have no specific cause that can be identified. Some people do seem to be more prone to forming stones than others, however. These include people who:

• do not drink enough fluids;
• have problems with urine that is static rather than draining through the urinary system as it should;
• have a urinary tract blockage;
• are unable to move around freely;
• have a medical condition that predisposes them to producing stones, such as a chronic UTI or an existing kidney disorder.

UNDER-8s

Children and bedwetting

During the first 2–3 years of life bedwetting at night is normal and expected, but by the age of five most children no longer urinate in their sleep. Bedwetting can be caused by the following:

• the child does not wake up when the bladder is full;
• there is an imbalance of the bladder muscles;
• the child has a small bladder;
• the child produces more urine than normal due to drinking too much before bed;
• low levels of ADH hormone;
• a urinary tract infection.

On rare occasions bedwetting can be caused by stress due to a major change, such as the birth of a sibling or parental separation. This can happen to children who have never had a bedwetting problem or who have been dry for some time.

Bedwetting can seriously affect a child's self-confidence, so lots of support should be given. Use plastic sheets, change the bed and child's nightwear calmly and quietly, and provide adequate night lighting so your child can reach the toilet easily. Most children grow out of the problem.

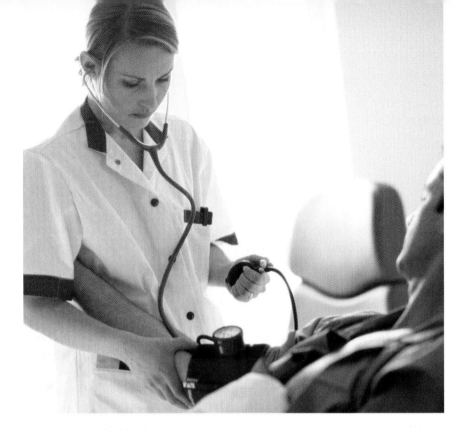

Blood pressure checks – how often?
Because hypertension is a warning sign of kidney disease, the over 40s should have their blood pressure checked at least every two years.

harmless, but they may not. If you have a problem with incontinence you do not need to suffer in silence: your doctor can refer you to a continence adviser for a thorough assessment. Once the results are available they will be able to advise on the best way to tackle the problem and improve the symptoms. Many symptoms of urinary problems are treatable.

WARNING SIGNS OF KIDNEY DISEASE

The following symptoms can signal a kidney problem:
- bloody or cloudy urine;
- foaming urine;
- puffiness of the eyes, hands or feet (especially in children);
- frequent night-time urination;
- high blood pressure.

Anyone with high blood pressure should have it checked regularly, as uncontrolled high blood pressure speeds kidney disease. Similarly, diabetes must be properly managed.

PROSTATE PROBLEMS

It is normal for the prostate gland in men to go through two major periods of growth. The first occurs at puberty, the second begins around the age of 25 and continues. This rarely causes problems in men under 40, but by the age of 60, most men will notice some symptoms of this continuing enlargement – usually the fact that the bladder does not empty properly, or it takes a long time to empty fully.

BLADDER CANCER

If you have repeated symptoms of bladder irritation – stinging, pain across the pubic bone, a need to urinate more frequently, and/or blood in your urine – it is important that your doctor tests your urine for cancer cells. If this is positive you should be referred to the local hospital's urology department for further investigation.

Sometimes the only symptoms of bladder cancer in the early stages are those of a UTI. The first visible sign is usually blood in the urine, though it can be that the blood is only seen in a urine test. Sometimes patients can be misdiagnosed as having a UTI and treated with antibiotics. However, though the symptoms may appear to improve, once the antibiotics are stopped the symptoms return.

BETTER SAFE THAN SORRY

If you think you have noticed that there has been an alteration in your bladder habits, discuss the changes with your GP. They may be

---

IT'S NOT TRUE!

'Incontinence only affects old people'

Contrary to popular belief, incontinence can affect anyone of any age, not just the elderly. Those mostly affected are women after childbirth and the menopause and men in later life, especially men with prostate problems.

The cost to the individual in terms of quality of life, loss of personal control and self-esteem is inestimable. It is therefore important that any incontinence problems are investigated to establish just what is causing the problem. Many people suffer in silence because incontinence is felt to be a 'taboo' subject. But attitudes are changing, and it is always worth seeing your doctor if you suffer (see pages 144–46).

The changes in pregnancy

A growing baby pressing on the bladder obviously causes significant changes in urinary habits. Knowing when these are normal, and how to cope when they are not, can make an enormous difference to your well-being at this time.

Changes in the body during pregnancy have an obvious effect on the urinary system. The added weight and pressure of pregnancy weakens the pelvic floor. The unborn baby pushes down on the bladder, the urethra and pelvic muscles. Temporary bladder control problems are common in pregnancy, and some can occur months or even years after childbirth. Exercising the pelvic floor (see pages 88–89) can help to prevent or minimise problems. However, changes in the position of the bladder and urethra, the stress of giving birth, having an episiotomy (when part of the perineum is cut to allow the baby to come through more easily), and any damage caused to the bladder control nerves during the birth can all change bladder function. Starting pelvic floor exercises as soon after the birth as possible can help to restore tone and normal function to the muscles.

PREGNANCY AND UTIs

Pregnant women are susceptible to UTIs for several reasons.

- The organs of the urinary tract become enlarged and dilated during pregnancy, leading to more urine being stored. When there is static urine in the system, bacteria are not flushed out as they should be, making infection more likely.
- During pregnancy a woman's urine contains greater than normal amounts of glucose and protein, which encourages bacteria to multiply.

- The automatic suppression of the immune system that enables the mother's body to tolerate the growing placenta and foetus can increase the risk of infection.
- A backflow of urine (from the bladder to the kidneys) is natural during pregnancy. This increases the likelihood of a UTI reaching the kidneys.

Why a UTI can be dangerous

Severe urinary tract and kidney infections pose a number of risks to the unborn child. Severe kidney infection makes a mother-to-be susceptible to septic shock, which can lead to cervical dilatation, the onset of early labour and all the resultant problems of a premature birth and baby.

A pregnant woman with a UTI is also more likely to develop a kidney infection. The high level of progesterone in the body relaxes the ureters, allowing urine to reflux back to the kidneys. Often the mother-to-be seeks help only when symptoms such as fever, chills, back pain and nausea set in, by which time she may already have a kidney infection.

Because of the risk to the unborn child, it is vital that a UTI is treated straightaway; the danger to the unborn child outweighs the danger of taking antibiotic drugs during pregnancy.

Weight control
Try to avoid putting on too much weight during pregnancy. Excess weight places additional stress on the bladder, which is already under pressure from the growing baby.

Adopting healthy habits

An unhealthy urinary system can make life miserable. Investing a little time and effort to make simple, healthy practices a habit will help to ensure that your bladder, urinary tract and kidneys stay trouble-free.

DRINK LOTS OF FLUID

The most important piece of advice that anyone could give you regarding your bladder is to drink plenty of fluid. You should drink at least two and preferably three litres of fluid a day; this may seem a great deal, but it is in fact a manageable amount – between 8 and 10 glasses a day.

Drinking this amount a day not only flushes the toxins out of your system, stimulating a sluggish metabolism, but flushes through the kidneys and bladder too. The more fluid you drink, the more urine is produced, so that you empty your bladder more frequently and toxins, including bacteria and parasites, are washed out of the body instead of sitting in the bladder. This should prevent them taking hold and causing an infection in the bladder or urinary tract.

Water is best

The majority of what you drink during the day should be water. Water has far fewer additives than fruit juices and commercially produced beverages such as tea, coffee, fruit drinks and cola drinks. In addition, some people find carbonated drinks or drinks with caffeine such as tea and coffee irritate the bladder, leading to symptoms such as a burning feeling when passing urine and/or a need to pass urine often.

BATHROOM HABITS

In general passing urine about once every three hours indicates a healthy bathroom habit. People who avoid passing urine for long periods of time are more likely to develop a urinary tract infection (UTI). They may also overstretch the bladder

muscle, causing it to lose tone, and in time they might lose the ability to empty the bladder completely. An empty bladder ensures that no stale urine containing toxins and bacteria has been left behind. To enable the bladder to empty properly, a woman should lean back against the wall or cistern behind her while sitting on the toilet seat.

Maintaining the highest standards of hygiene will also lessen the chances of developing a UTI. To ensure bacteria are moved away from the urethral opening, a woman in particular should always wipe from front to back after a bowel movement. And if she needs to touch her urethra, she should always make sure to wash her hands beforehand.

FROM THE OUTSIDE IN

An irritated bladder becomes sore and more vulnerable to bacteria. Anyone prone to irritation and UTIs should find that keeping external irritants to a minimum will help. Soaps, bubble bath lotions, deodorants, biological soap powders

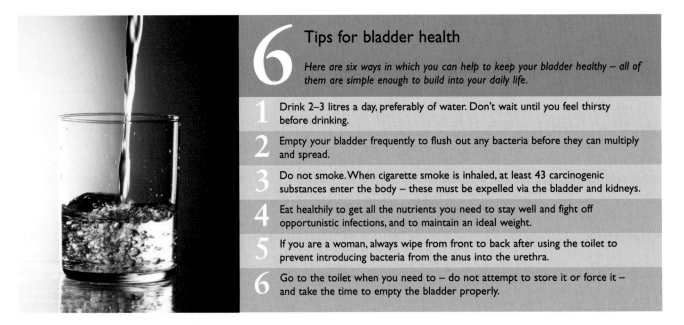

6 Tips for bladder health

Here are six ways in which you can help to keep your bladder healthy – all of them are simple enough to build into your daily life.

1 Drink 2–3 litres a day, preferably of water. Don't wait until you feel thirsty before drinking.

2 Empty your bladder frequently to flush out any bacteria before they can multiply and spread.

3 Do not smoke. When cigarette smoke is inhaled, at least 43 carcinogenic substances enter the body – these must be expelled via the bladder and kidneys.

4 Eat healthily to get all the nutrients you need to stay well and fight off opportunistic infections, and to maintain an ideal weight.

5 If you are a woman, always wipe from front to back after using the toilet to prevent introducing bacteria from the anus into the urethra.

6 Go to the toilet when you need to – do not attempt to store it or force it – and take the time to empty the bladder properly.

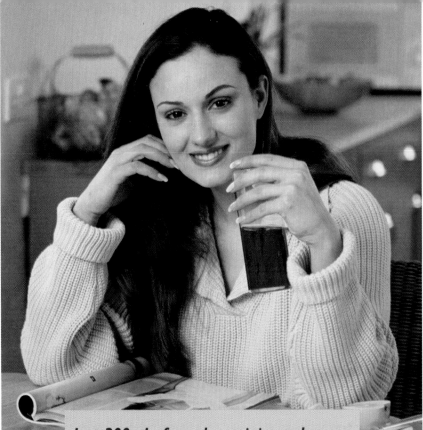

Just 300ml of cranberry juice a day can significantly lower the risk of cystitis, according to one US study.

for washing clothes and the chemicals in bathroom cleaners can all irritate the urethra and bladder. Some people are irritated by dyes used in coloured toilet paper. During menstruation, it is wise for a woman to change a tampon each time she passes urine. Prolonged activities such as cycling or horseriding may irritate the urethral area; in addition, the clothing worn during these activities is often tight and restrictive, which keeps the urethral area warm and moist, and more receptive to bacteria.

EAT A HEALTHY DIET

Eating five servings of fresh fruit and vegetables a day, as recommended by dietitians, also helps when it comes to keeping your bladder healthy.

Research shows that eating certain vegetables regularly – especially carrots and tomatoes – can reduce your chances of developing bladder or prostate cancer.

CRANBERRY JUICE

Some people find that drinking cranberry juice helps to prevent urinary infection. This is often thought to be because the cranberry makes the urine more acidic and therefore more difficult for bacteria to survive in. However, it is more likely to be the fact that there is a substance in cranberries that prevents bacteria adhering to the side of the bladder, so they are flushed out when you pass urine.

If you find the taste of cranberry juice too sharp, try cranberry capsules instead; these are available in health food shops. Another alternative is to drink the mixed

cranberry juices that are available, although these are not as effective as pure cranberry juice.

KEEP YOUR WEIGHT UNDER CONTROL

Being significantly overweight is undoubtedly bad for your health, and the bladder and kidneys are among those organs most seriously affected by excess weight.

- Obese people run a greater risk of developing high blood pressure, diabetes, cardiovascular disease, endocrine abnormalities, lung problems and arthritis. Diabetes and high blood pressure are leading causes of kidney failure.

- Being overweight puts a strain on the pelvic floor and bladder, and so may contribute to incontinence.

- A very obese person who is unable to move about easily may have problems using normal

Watch your weight

Obesity can cause a range of urinary problems. An enlarged abdomen pressing against the bladder can weaken the bladder valve, causing urine leakage.

Smoking and bladder cancer

The majority of cases of bladder cancer are triggered by external factors such as smoking. In fact, smoking causes one in two of all cases of bladder cancer. Harmful chemicals – often originating in cigarettes or used in industry – can trigger cancerous cell changes in the inside wall of the bladder. Cancer of the bladder most usually strikes people between the ages of 60 and 80. More common in men than women, it is one of the most common forms of cancer for men.

It is never too late to stop smoking. Research shows that people who have stopped, even if they smoked for several decades, are less likely to get bladder cancer than those who continue to smoke.

CONTROLLING IC

Interstitial cystitis (IC) is a chronic inflammation of the bladder wall, with symptoms similar to those of a UTI. Doctors do not know what causes it – it may be caused by an autoimmune response or a specific gene – so currently all treatments are aimed at relieving symptoms.

In addition to following general guidelines for good bladder health, people should try to identify what triggers their symptoms. Many foods and drinks have been found by some people to cause or aggravate IC, these include:

- alcohol
- chocolate
- tomatoes

- spices
- caffeine
- artificial sweeteners

By cutting out these substances then reintroducing them one by one it may be possible to identify a culprit. Often people find it helpful to keep a 'voiding diary' to monitor the frequency and times of urination.

Exercise helps some people, while others benefit from bladder training, which involves emptying the bladder at designated times only – the use of relaxation techniques and distractions can also help with this.

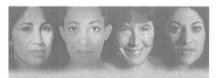

SEX AND URINARY HEALTH

Women who are prone to urinary tract infections may find it helpful to follow these simple rules before and after sex:

- Both partners should wash their hands and genitals just before sex takes place.
- Use lubrication during sex to reduce any urethral irritation.
- Urinate about 10 minutes after sex to flush out bacteria, and wash again.
- Choose contraception with care: inserting a diaphragm, for example, can introduce bacteria and it can press on the bladder, making it difficult to pee effectively.

If sex is infrequent but inevitably results in cystitis, the doctor may recommend taking low dose post-coital antibiotics.

bathroom and toilet facilities, which may make toilet hygiene and continence difficult.
- Recent research shows that obese people are at a greater risk of developing certain cancers – for example, overweight men have a higher than average mortality rate from prostate, kidney and colorectal cancer.

DON'T SMOKE

Smoking cigarettes can damage your kidneys and urinary system in several ways. Smoking is a contributory factor towards narrowing of the arteries, which often leads to high blood pressure: both conditions are potentially harmful to kidneys. Chronic coughing can worsen any problems with bladder control – the extra pressure causes urine leakage.

Sleep on your back
Some research suggests that sleeping on the stomach increases the risk of kidney stones.

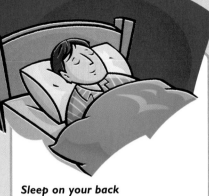

Eat smaller amounts of protein
Smaller amounts of protein mean less uric acid, calcium and oxalate carried in urine, making stones less likely.

Drink more fluids
This will flush more unwanted waste products out of the kidneys. But be aware that vitamin C, including cranberry juice, can make urine more acidic and increase the chances of producing uric acid or cystine stones. On the other hand, milk and citrus fruits can make urine more alkaline and increase the chances of producing calcium phosphate stones. Water is the best choice of fluids.

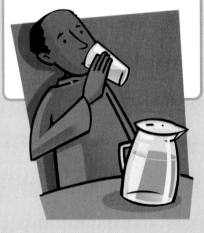

AVOIDING KIDNEY STONES

Kidney stones affect more men than women, and some common stones result from metabolic disorders which are inherited. However if you – or any of your family members – have a history of kidney stones, these guidelines may help prevent a recurrence.

Eat fewer oxalate-rich foods
Beans, soft fruits, spinach and chocolate should be avoided if you have had an oxalate-rich stone.

Increase your fibre intake
Eat more fruit and vegetables, whole grains and wholemeal bread.

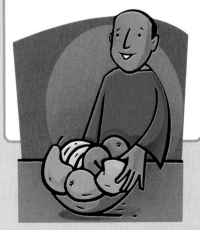

Eat less salt
Salt and salty foods increase the amount of calcium in the urine, which contributes to the commonest types of kidney stones.

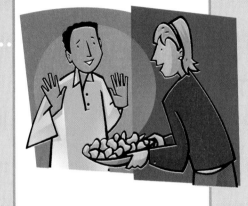

Don't overdo antacids
Some diuretics and antacids may increase the amount of calcium in urine, which can lead to stones forming.

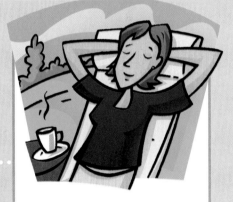

Learn to relax
There is an association between stress and kidney stones.

The right clothes

The kind of clothing you wear has more impact than you might imagine on the health of your bladder and urinary tract. What you wear is especially important if you are prone to urinary tract infections.

DRESSING FOR BLADDER HEALTH

Certain fabrics are better for bladder health than others. It's best to wear fabrics made from natural fibres, preferably 100 per cent cotton or silk, especially if you are susceptible to urinary tract infections. Natural fibres such as cotton allow the skin to breathe and are also very absorbent. Wearing 100 per cent cotton ensures that the area around the urethra remains dry, rather than becoming moist and irritated. You should not wear nylon underwear – and nylon pants with a cotton gusset have not been found to be an effective alternative to those which are all cotton.

It is also important that underwear and trousers fit comfortably and are not too tight. Any item of clothing that is too tight will rub and irritate the groin area and contribute to a build-up of heat and moisture.

Women prone to urinary tract infections should not wear tights, leggings or trousers too often. Wearing a skirt and, weather permitting, going bare legged allows air to circulate so there is less chance of a moist, warm environment developing which would encourage bacteria to reproduce and migrate up the

The hidden culprit?
Washing powder is often overlooked as a source of irritation. Changing to a non-biological powder and double rinsing underwear could reduce the frequency and severity of urinary infections.

urethra into the bladder, causing an infection which could potentially spread to the kidneys.

BE LAUNDRY WISE

Washing powders can be another source of irritation. Just as you should stop using scented bath or shower products if these cause an infection, biological soap powders should be avoided. Irritation occurs when skin is in contact with chemical residues on the material.

Whatever the washing powder or liquid used, it's important that clothes are thoroughly rinsed afterwards to remove the powder residue. If in any doubt, put clothes through the rinse cycle twice.

Wash clothes – especially underwear – with the water heated to a temperature of at least 60°C, to kill off any bacteria in the fabric fibres. Luckily, cotton and linen are better able to withstand washing in hotter water than many man-made fibres. Washing items in water heated to 40°C may not kill all the bacteria. And any bacteria remaining are likely to become active again the next time the item of clothing is worn, and consequently warmed up.

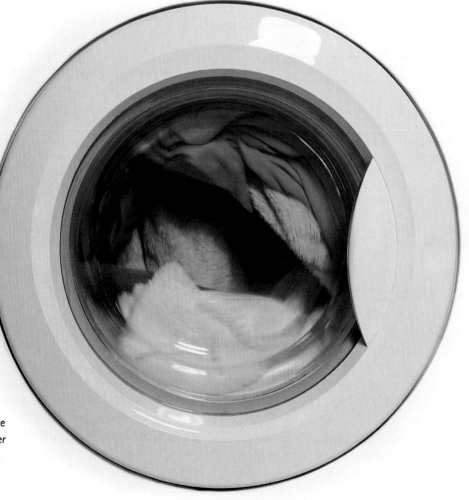

PROTECTING THE KIDNEYS

The kidneys are vulnerable to harm from two basic external sources: from a trauma or blow, and from the cold. In both cases, there is a lot you can do to protect yourself.

Sports

Boxers and those who play contact sports such as ice hockey, wear a special protective belt that shields the kidneys from stray blows. In motorcycle racing and other fast, potentially dangerous sports such as snowboarding, people wear padded clothing and special support belts that help to protect the kidneys and lower back in case of trauma.

The cold and your kidneys

Kidneys can be affected by cold exposure and so should be well protected with warm layers of clothing. Despite this fact and the well-known saying, you cannot 'catch a chill' in your kidneys. People sometimes feel an invasion of cold in their back when they are exposed to wind, cold or damp, but it is more likely that the sensations they experience are caused by the kidneys responding to the body's falling core temperature. This is particularly noticeable in cases of hypothermia.

Hypothermia is defined as having a core body temperature of less than 35°C (95°F). Cases are not confined to winter: it can happen even in summer if you swim too long in cold water, or are exposed to high winds. When a person has hypothermia, the body diverts blood from the extremities in order to keep the vital organs – heart, brain, liver and kidneys – working effectively. As the body's core temperature falls, the kidneys extract more fluid from the

bloodstream and this increases urine production. In addition, chilled kidneys are less able to retain fluids which is why nearly all victims of hypothermia are dehydrated. Other signs of hypothermia include:
- cold hands and feet;
- mental confusion;
- sluggishness and lethargy.

If you suspect someone is suffering from hypothermia:
- protect them from the wind;
- give warm drinks, and avoid alcohol and coffee;
- make sure they change into dry layered clothes;
- apply heat to the kidney area: blood circulates through the kidneys every two minutes and heat improves the flow;
- add plenty of layers – a sleeping bag is ideal;
- make sure they urinate frequently, a full bladder is a site of heat loss.

What you don't do is also important. Improving blood flow to the extremities is not an immediate priority as this diverts blood from the vital organs. This should be done once the core temperature has been raised. Similarly, do not elevate someone's legs (the standard treatment for shock) as this puts cold blood back into the circulation.

Anyone who has existing kidney problems or diabetes should be aware that these conditions increase the risk of hypothermia, and take every precaution when outdoors in poor weather conditions.

UNDER-10s

Winter fun and cold awareness

Playing outdoors in the winter is great fun for children, but it is important to protect their kidneys by following a few simple points.
- **Layers** Children should be dressed warmly in at least three layers to trap heat next to the body. A vest or close-fitting teeshirt next to the skin, a warm layer such as fleece and a wind-proof top layer are a good start.
- **Time limits** Set limits for how long children spend outdoors, and have frequent indoor breaks so they can warm up. Children often don't notice how cold they are when they are distracted.
- **Hot drinks** Fluid lost through perspiration should be replaced: hot drinks also help to increase the body's core temperature.
- **Warming up** Get them out of wet clothes as soon as possible and change them into something warm and loose fitting. If they are still cold, they should have a warm bath or cuddle a warm hot water bottle to the kidney area.
- **Safety** When sledging, children should not lie flat, as this increases the risk of abdominal injuries.

Be aware of environmental hazards

Pollutants that pose a threat to the kidneys and bladder include lead, asbestos and aromatic amines. These toxins are silent, invisible and can be deadly. They are taken in with the air we breathe, the water we drink and the food we eat.

LEAD AND THE KIDNEYS

The accumulation of lead within the body can cause kidney damage and even kidney failure, as well as high blood pressure. Recent research suggests that even low levels of lead in the body are harmful to health.

The dangers of lead poisoning

Lead particles are found in oil-based paint, water that has passed through lead piping, contaminated soil, and leaded petrol exhaust fumes.

For adults, the risk of lead poisoning is low, but lead poisoning remains one of the most common and devastating environmental diseases among children. Young children are likely to put things into their mouths that have been in contact with lead-contaminated paint, dust or soil. In addition, children absorb 50 per cent of any lead they inhale or swallow, whereas adults absorb only 10 per cent.

Ingested lead is mistaken for calcium by the body, and cannot be broken down into a substance which can be removed from the body. As a result, it is permanently absorbed into the bones and the brain.

The effects of lead poisoning are varied, long-term and potentially fatal. They include kidney disease, heart disease and strokes. The accumulation of lead in the brain of a growing child, in the past from leaded petrol, can result in learning disabilities, speech and language handicaps, behavioural problems neurological defects and lowered IQ.

LEAD AND YOUR HOME

Any building constructed before 1960 may have lead paint in it somewhere. All surfaces – wood, metal or plaster – coated with paint containing lead are potential health hazards. Posing the greatest risks are:
- Surfaces in poor condition, that are peeling, chipped or flaking.
- Surfaces that have been disturbed, as when a house is renovated.
- Surfaces within reach of children, such as door frames, skirting boards, railings, window-sills or painted radiators.

PROTECTING YOUR FAMILY

There are various simple precautions you can take to protect your family from environmental risk factors. Although for most people most of the time, the risk to health from toxins in the home and workplace is small, it is worth taking steps to protect yourself.

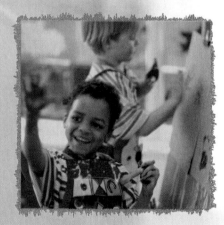

CHOOSE PAINTS WISELY
Aromatic amines are found in artists' materials including children's fingerpaints. There is little evidence that these pose a risk to child health but it may be wise to avoid products containing 2-naphthylamine, 4-chloro-o-toluidine and 4-amino-biphenyls.

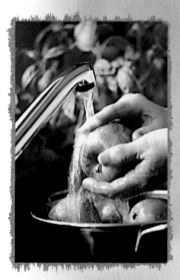

FRUIT FOR HEALTH
Washing all fruit and vegetables before eating them can reduce the amount of lead you ingest: this is particularly important for children.

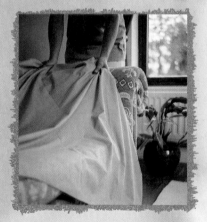

PROTECT AND COVER
Old houses may still contain significant amounts of lead paint, even if it has been overpainted several times. When stripping paint, use protective clothes, a mask and dust sheets.

- Any surfaces that are subject to friction or abrasion, such as windows, doors or floors.

Lead poisoning is preventable. A few simple precautions can help to prevent you and your children ingesting dust lead particles at home.

- Always wash your hands before preparing or eating food.
- Wash fruit and vegetables.
- Wash your hands whenever you come indoors, especially if you have been in contact with sand, soil or a pet.
- Wash children's toys frequently.
- Don't smoke. Cigarettes contain lead: a smoker who lives in a dust-laden environment will have higher levels of lead in their blood than a non-smoker.

If you have reason to suspect that your home was once decorated with lead-based paint:

- Consider fitting wooden or washable floor coverings, instead of carpets. Vacuuming, sweeping and dusting release any lead particles trapped in carpets and soft furnishings into the air.
- After dusting and vacuuming, allow dust to settle for an hour, then wipe down all surfaces with a wet cloth or mop. Add a little sugar soap to the water you use; it contains high levels of phosphate detergents, which are very efficient at picking up lead particles.

Lead and nutrition

More lead is absorbed when ingested on an empty stomach, and when calcium and iron levels within the body are low. This is especially true for children, who should be encouraged to eat frequent meals and snacks, and to enjoy a balanced diet,

high in calcium, iron, zinc, vitamin C and protein, and low in high-fat foods. Foods rich in iron and vitamin C include lean meat, eggs, raisins, green vegetables, fruit, milk, cheese and potatoes.

Lead and the workplace

Anyone who works in an environment which exposes them to lead is at risk of lead poisoning, as is anyone who has a hobby that brings them into contact with lead, such as pottery, restoring old furniture or fishing. Many garages and sheds have lead in their environment.

Lead-laden dust can contaminate work clothes and shoes. Launder work clothes separately or better still away from your home, using a phosphate detergent, which will remove more lead particles from the fabric than other washing powders.

TOYS TO GUM
Many PVC toys contain lead and cadmium which can leach out when children 'gum' them. Consumer groups are targeting toy companies to get such products withdrawn.

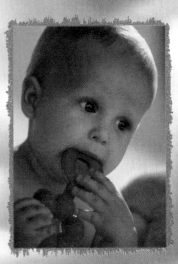

FILTER DRINKING WATER
If you have any reason to suspect contamination from lead or aromatic amines, filter your drinking water.

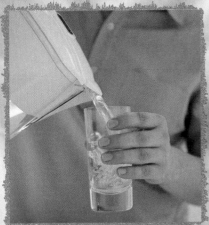

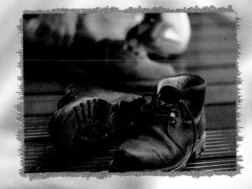

OUTDOOR SHOES
Remove shoes outdoors if you can to avoid treading lead into the home.

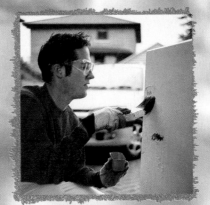

PROTECT YOURSELF
Strict regulations are in place to protect those working in hazardous industries: take every precaution indicated in your company's safety policy.

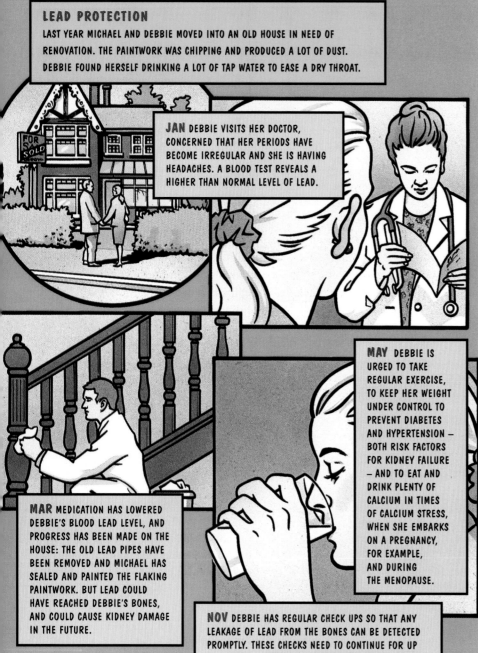

LEAD PROTECTION
LAST YEAR MICHAEL AND DEBBIE MOVED INTO AN OLD HOUSE IN NEED OF RENOVATION. THE PAINTWORK WAS CHIPPING AND PRODUCED A LOT OF DUST. DEBBIE FOUND HERSELF DRINKING A LOT OF TAP WATER TO EASE A DRY THROAT.

JAN DEBBIE VISITS HER DOCTOR, CONCERNED THAT HER PERIODS HAVE BECOME IRREGULAR AND SHE IS HAVING HEADACHES. A BLOOD TEST REVEALS A HIGHER THAN NORMAL LEVEL OF LEAD.

MAR MEDICATION HAS LOWERED DEBBIE'S BLOOD LEAD LEVEL, AND PROGRESS HAS BEEN MADE ON THE HOUSE: THE OLD LEAD PIPES HAVE BEEN REMOVED AND MICHAEL HAS SEALED AND PAINTED THE FLAKING PAINTWORK. BUT LEAD COULD HAVE REACHED DEBBIE'S BONES, AND COULD CAUSE KIDNEY DAMAGE IN THE FUTURE.

MAY DEBBIE IS URGED TO TAKE REGULAR EXERCISE, TO KEEP HER WEIGHT UNDER CONTROL TO PREVENT DIABETES AND HYPERTENSION – BOTH RISK FACTORS FOR KIDNEY FAILURE – AND TO EAT AND DRINK PLENTY OF CALCIUM IN TIMES OF CALCIUM STRESS, WHEN SHE EMBARKS ON A PREGNANCY, FOR EXAMPLE, AND DURING THE MENOPAUSE.

NOV DEBBIE HAS REGULAR CHECK UPS SO THAT ANY LEAKAGE OF LEAD FROM THE BONES CAN BE DETECTED PROMPTLY. THESE CHECKS NEED TO CONTINUE FOR UP TO 20 YEARS TO BE SURE THERE IS NO KIDNEY DAMAGE.

ASBESTOS AND THE KIDNEYS

Breathing in asbestos fibres not only causes lung cancer, but also increases the risk of cancer of the kidneys, stomach, oesophagus and pancreas.

Kidney cancer accounts for about two per cent of all cancer cases, and is twice as common in men as in women. The causes of kidney cancer are not fully understood, but asbestos, along with tobacco and cadmium (found chiefly in batteries, molten metals, cigarette smoke and cadmium-contaminated food) are among the carcinogens responsible.

Asbestos was used in the construction of all kinds of buildings, including many homes. In industry, it was found to be an ideal heat-resistant fabric for coating or packaging tubes and pipes, for instance, and a key component in the making of brake and transmission parts for cars.

When is asbestos dangerous?

Airborne or waterborne asbestos fibres do not disperse, evaporate or dissolve, hence their danger. Asbestos dust in the air can be inhaled, or eaten or swallowed with food or drink. Asbestos can enter drinking water if the system is fitted with pipes made of asbestos cement.

Who is at risk?

People who come into contact with asbestos dust in the workplace or while renovating or demolishing buildings fitted with asbestos are most at risk of health problems. However, regulations introduced in the 1970s have made working with asbestos in industry much safer than it was in the past. Asbestos is now bonded with other materials or encased, so that handlers are much less likely to inhale the toxic dust.

AROMATIC AMINES

Aromatic amines are chemicals used to produce dyes, plastics, pesticides and other products. Direct links between the dye industry and bladder cancer were established as long ago as the 19th century and, as a result, the synthetic dye industry in the USA was shut down in the 1970s. However, workers are still being exposed to these substances, as production has since moved to developing countries with less stringent safety practices.

Since they are highly soluble, aromatic amines can find their way into the water supply and travel far from the point of contamination. Contaminated water may have an unpleasant odour; if you suspect that there may be aromatic amines in your water supply, the water can be tested for traces of this toxin.

Drugs and the kidneys

The active ingredients in the medications we take are broken down in the liver and removed by the kidneys. If the kidneys are impaired, drugs may remain in the system longer than intended, which can affect the way they act on our bodies.

TAKING MEDICATION SAFELY

It is important to remember that any drug you take – be it prescribed or obtained over the counter – is a powerful medication designed to alter the way your body works. Whatever the circumstances – whether you have problems with your kidneys or liver, or if you simply want to stay safe and avoid problems in the future – it is vital that before you take any drug you know the correct dose and how it should be taken. Using medication improperly, taking too much or too little, or combining it with other drugs or alcohol, can put you at risk.

The effects of ageing

As we age, liver and kidney functions slow down, and take longer to process and excrete any drugs we have taken. In addition, the percentage of water and muscle in the body usually decreases and the percentage of body fat increases. These changes can alter how long it takes for a drug to be absorbed into the body, how much of the drug is actually absorbed and how long the drug remains in the body before it is excreted. As a result, the same drugs can act differently on the body from when we were younger.

Knowing how the drug works
It is important to know when to take medication – whether before or after a meal, if there are any foods that you should avoid, and whether it is safe to drink alcohol while on the medication.

Multiple drug prescriptions

The situation is complicated for many patients by the fact that they have been prescribed more than one drug. For example, a patient may be taking a drug to control bladder spasms while also taking an antibiotic for a UTI, and maybe a painkiller as well. In addition, medication for an underlying disease such as high blood pressure or a cardiac problem may be prescribed. All these drugs interact not only with the body, but also with each other. This increases the possibility of experiencing an unwanted drug reaction or of over-medication.

Antibiotics increase the risk of urinary tract infections

TALKING POINT

Taking prescribed antibiotics, for whatever reason, can lead to bacteria in your body gradually becoming resistant to them, especially if you take antibiotics every time you have a flare-up of infection. This is because antibiotics kill the bacteria that are susceptible to them, leaving behind those that are resistant. In time, the majority of bacteria of a particular strain can become resistant to a particular group of antibiotics. Stronger and stronger antibiotics will be needed, until the danger is that bacteria will emerge which will simply not respond to any antibiotics at all. For this reason, a doctor will only prescribe antibiotics that are necessary.

A billion dollars' worth of antibiotics are prescribed for UTIs in the USA each year.

Before taking any medication you should be aware of the following:
- How the drug works.
- Whether it reacts with any other drugs that you are taking.
- The correct dosage and when and how it should be taken.
- That you must finish taking the entire course prescribed for you.
- If you experience unexpected side effects, don't just stop – consult your doctor.

ACCIDENTAL DRUG MISUSE
Older people sometimes require hospital treatment as a result of incorrectly using prescription and/or over-the-counter drugs. A patient is sometimes on a variety of medications without even their GP being aware of all the precise details. They may be under more than one specialist, each of whom has prescribed drugs for different problems without an exact knowledge of what other drugs the patient is also taking.

Don't overuse antibiotics
Using antibiotics too often to combat urinary tract infections (UTIs) can lead to bacteria in the bladder and urinary tract gradually becoming resistant to the antibiotics. Therefore it's best to take antibiotics only when you have an acute infection – this will ensure that when you do need antibiotics, they will do the job.

If your only symptoms are urine smelling a little different than usual and a bit of discomfort in the bladder area, and you otherwise feel well, you may be able to treat an infection by following the general rules for good bladder health (see pages 48–50), drinking plenty of water, resting and applying a hot water bottle over the kidneys, without resorting to antibiotics.

However, if symptoms are more severe – your urine has blood in it, you experience fever and chills, painful kidneys and/or general flu-like symptoms – it is important that you take a specimen of urine to your doctor for analysis and take any antibiotics prescribed to treat the infection. Always finish a course of tablets to ensure the infection clears completely.

Safety with antidepressants
Think carefully before taking any antidepressants, if you also have a UTI. Drugs such as Prozac or Imipramine may prevent the bladder from contracting properly, so that it is never fully emptied. The resulting static urine can cause repeated urine infection, and the only way to empty the bladder may prove to be by using a catheter.

HERBAL REMEDIES
Some herbal remedies are reputed to be helpful when dealing with kidney and bladder complaints, but keep in mind they are not regulated by any official medical body. The assumption is that because herbal remedies are 'natural', they are not harmful in any way. In a notorious case in Belgium in the 1990s, more than 100 women developed kidney disease after taking Chinese herbs prescribed by a weight reduction clinic. These women needed dialysis or a kidney transplant, and some went on to develop bladder cancer.

45-60 YEARS

Why topical oestrogen replacement may be good for your urinary system

The menopause in women leads, amongst other things, to changes in the pelvic floor, bladder and genital area. The walls of the urethra and the lower bladder become thinner, blood flow is reduced, the elasticity of the connective tissue decreases and the muscles begin to shrivel. Women going through these changes are more likely than before to experience problems with UTIs, difficulties with emptying the bladder, and incontinence. However, some relief from these symptoms can be gained with hormone replacement therapy (HRT). Replacing the oestrogen lost during the menopause, either by taking tablets or by using topical creams or vaginal pessaries, reverses these changes. Using a topical product has the advantage that symptoms in the specific area can be dealt with in the first instance. But changes do not occur overnight. It may take at least a month to see any improvement and 6–12 months for things to settle completely.

Before embarking on a herbal remedy, you should check it out with your doctor or pharmacist. It is particularly important to check that any remedies you are interested in can be safely combined with any prescription or over-the-counter drugs that you are also taking.

BE KIDNEY WISE TO OTC MEDICATIONS

The many over-the-counter (OTC) medications that are available are harmless to most individuals when used correctly. However, recent research suggests that some of the most popular OTC medications are not safe to take if you have any problems with the health of your kidneys. Those with kidney disease are more at risk of developing problems with OTC medicines, due to their often-complex medical condition and multiple drug therapy.

OTC products require careful assessment before their use by anyone with a kidney ailment. At the very least you should read medication labels and any accompanying leaflets carefully. If in any doubt at all, consult your doctor about which OTC drugs are safe.

Beware OTC painkillers

Chronic kidney damage caused by taking over-the-counter painkillers over a long period of time accounts for 5–30 per cent of patients referred for dialysis or kidney transplant worldwide. The good news is that if the user stops taking the painkillers the condition of the damaged kidneys often stabilises – sometimes even improves. On the other hand, a continued intake of painkillers progressively worsens the kidney damage.

HERBS FOR BLADDER AND KIDNEY FUNCTION?

If you are planning to try a herbal remedy, remember that there are no regulations governing herbalists in the UK. In addition, doctors who specialise in kidney disease are wary of herbal medication because its results can cause lasting damage.

DIURETIC HERBS
These increase urine production. They include dandelion leaf, artichoke, bitter/sweet apple, broom, corn silk, juniper, onion, parsley, cleavers, yarrow, and hydrangea root.

CORN SILK
Is reputed to soothe tissues and protect the inflamed urinary tract.

WHITE WILLOW
A mild natural analgesic (a drug that relieves pain).

UVA URSI
This is claimed to be an antiseptic, to help to dissolve kidney stones, and also to be effective against bedwetting.

SAW PALMETTO
Reputed to reduce inflammation and pain in the prostate.

HORSE AND BURDOCK
These are both said to nourish the urinary system.

The painkillers most likely to damage the kidneys are those that combine two or more different analgesics, such as aspirin plus paracetamol. This can increase the toxicity of each analgesic, and they often contain caffeine or codeine (or both) as well, which can sometimes prove to be addictive.

If you are taking over-the-counter painkillers on a regular basis, be sure to check with your doctor that they are not damaging your kidneys. This is particularly vital if you already have any kind of kidney disorder.

Who should not take NSAIDs

Nonsteroidal anti-inflammatory drugs (NSAIDs) – most notably aspirin and ibuprofen – are taken to ease all sorts of pain, and are so easy to buy that you even find them in supermarkets. Unfortunately, they irritate the stomach lining and this, together with other side effects, suggests that anyone who suffers from reduced kidney function, ulcers, Crohn's disease, asthma or has blood clotting problems would be unwise to take them. Although medical research in the USA has indicated that there does not seem to be any 'significant associations' between these tablets and kidney failure, scientists in the UK are more cautious. They would not recommend taking these drugs if you have kidney damage.

Why paracetamol may be safer

Paracetamol is thought to be safer to take than NSAIDs if you have any problems with your kidneys. This is because it works in a different way from aspirin and other NSAIDs. Paracetamol works mainly on receptors in the brain, while aspirin – for example – works on similar receptors throughout the body. So paracetamol can dull pain and reduce fever without interfering with other body systems.

STREET DRUGS AND THE KIDNEYS

Illegal drugs such as ecstasy, crack, cocaine, speed and heroin can seriously damage the kidneys and urinary system. This is due to the direct effect of toxic substances in the body (which the kidneys must eliminate) and indirect reactions that can lead to impaired kidney function and kidney failure. As a result, drug-users can require lifelong dialysis or kidney transplant.

Ecstasy, for example, can cause dehydration, hyperthermia and heatstroke. Although people may react by drinking more water, ecstasy also triggers the release of ADH, causing urinary retention. This results in 'water intoxication' (see page 63), which can cause a swelling of the brain, and lead to coma or death.

In 2000, the number of deaths in the UK relating to ecstasy use exceeded the number of road traffic deaths in 15–24 year olds.

Pure pleasure
Clubbing has become linked in people's minds with drug use, but it's important to remember that thousands enjoy dancing without taking dangerous substances.

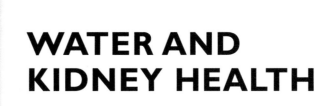

WATER AND KIDNEY HEALTH

Our bodies are mostly water. Up to two-thirds of body weight is water. Everything we do – from drawing a breath to running a marathon – has an impact on the amount of water in the body. This section explains why we need water, how we get it and how our bodies use it.

 62 *The body normally balances the water it loses with thirst so the water you drink is enough to keep the urinary system working efficiently.*

 65 *Find out why water is the best drink for health, and follow our tips on how to get more water into your daily life.*

 69 *Dehydration means the body does not have enough water and causes sluggishness and poor concentration. Learn how to prevent this.*

Why do we need water?

One of the basic principles of all living things is the need to maintain constant concentrations of all the chemicals which enable cells to function. Water is essential in the processes that maintain this equilibrium.

Life developed initially in water, so physiological structures and processes were needed to keep out excess water which would otherwise dilute the composition of the living cells. As a broad generalisation, the human body starts to malfunction if there is a 5 per cent excess of water. Vital organs may be critically damaged and both physical and mental functions are seriously affected by a 5–10 per cent dilution of body fluids by water.

When life emerged on to dry land, the opposite problem, dehydration, became a possibility. As another generalisation, organ functions and physical and mental performance are adversely affected by a 2–5 per cent loss of water, and critically affected by 10 per cent dehydration.

Water forms a large proportion of our bodies – around 60–80 per cent by weight. The exact proportion for individuals varies depending on body weight: fat contains no water, so the more fat a person carries, the lower the percentage of water in the body. The amount of water is difficult to measure exactly, but what is more important is fluctuation and that is easily measured by noting changes in body weight. The body works best, in terms of function and performance, over a narrow range of variation in terms of water content.

LOSING WATER

We are constantly losing water, in urine, in sweat, and as vapour in our breath. The amount being lost varies under the influence of environmental conditions, physical activity, food and drink consumed and any medication being taken. It is therefore necessary to drink at different rates in order to match the losses from the body, and this gives rise to the concept of 'fluid balance'.

Under usual climatic conditions, and without physical activity, we lose about 500ml a day in sweat and in breath. Another 100–200ml or so is lost from the bowel in stools, and it is necessary to pass at least 750ml as urine to keep the kidneys functioning properly and remove toxic waste products of metabolism. So for health, in round terms, we need to consume a minimum of about 1.5 litres (2½ pints) of water daily, in drinks and in foods. The absolute minimum varies from person to person, mainly according to size, but it is difficult to establish a definitive minimum for any individual.

Humans can survive without food for some weeks, but die after only 2–3 days without water: babies, breastfeeding mothers and the elderly may not even survive this long without water.

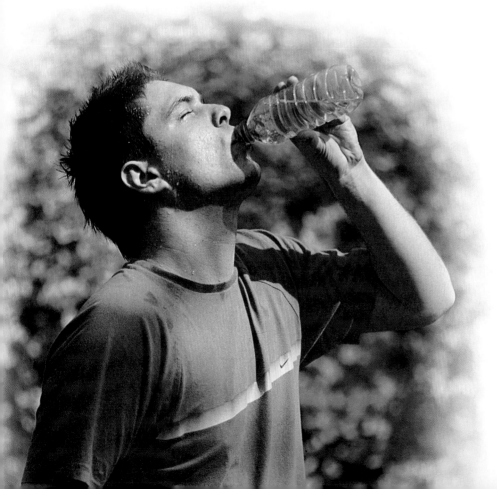

Balancing acts
Working up a sweat during exercise means your body needs to take in more water than the usually recommended 8–10 glasses a day. Not replacing lost fluids can lead to muscle cramps, confusion and even coma.

'You can't drink too much water'

A healthy person has to drink a lot to develop 'water intoxication', but it can occur more easily in infants or children. A few years ago, some diabetic children developed epileptic seizures: the artificial sweeteners in sugar-free drinks were blamed, but the answer ultimately seemed to be the volume of liquid these children were drinking – 2 or 3 litres at a time. Large volumes of beer might produce water intoxication in adults, as could any drink consumed in greater quantities than the limit of the kidneys' filtration rate – about 1–2 litres an hour.

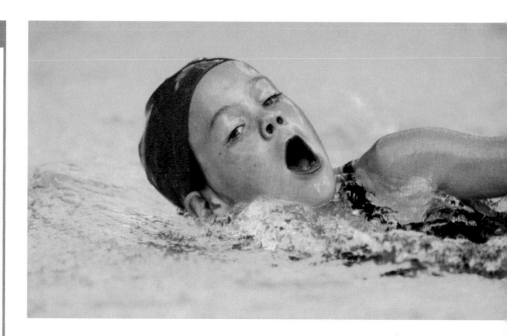

However, it would be dangerous to drink this amount under normal conditions, because it exceeds the maximum capacity of the kidneys to excrete excess water, leading to a state of 'water intoxication'.

Waterlogging the system
Prolonged swimming is said to cause small children to take in excessive water and water intoxication can result. Water intoxication lowers the concentration of salt in the body, resulting in lethargy, confusion and coma.

WHAT AFFECTS FLUID BALANCE?

The minimum water consumption necessary to achieve fluid balance varies with physical size. Larger people have a greater skin area so produce more sweat, and also have higher metabolic rates, so they require more oxygen and food. They thus need to breathe more, so more water evaporates in the breath. Therefore larger people need to drink more, particularly when exercising.

In hot dry temperatures, which cause more rapid water evaporation from the skin and lungs, and at high levels of physical activity, healthy people can lose water at a rate of up to 1.5 litres an hour. In certain conditions, therefore, some people might need up to 20 litres of water a day to avoid dehydration.

FLUID RETENTION

Fluid retention, or oedema, is a common condition. It is potentially serious in anyone who displays other signs of kidney, liver or heart disease.

On the other hand, mild oedema – swelling of ankles or extremities – is a common reaction to a variety of stresses, and of no great consequence. The commonest cause is obesity which retards the return of blood from the legs, so fluid accumulates. Oedema also develops after muscle injuries, muscle use, or sitting or standing for extended periods. Some women experience oedema as part of premenstrual syndrome.

The solution to mild fluid retention of this kind is to deal with its cause: to lose weight (if overweight), or to become more physically active while taking steps to avoid muscle damage.

Diuretic medications

Most diuretic medications work by removing sodium (salt) from the body, on the premise that water will follow the salt. This is only recommended, and only safe, when for medical reasons the body has accumulated excess sodium, usually as a result of heart problems or serious kidney disease.

Herbal preparations

Many herbs are reputed to treat fluid retention, particularly for menstruating women. While most are probably safe, consult your doctor if you experience severe fluid retention as part of premenstrual syndrome.

Diuretics do not help weight loss: they promote the loss of water, salt and potassium – rather than fat – from the body.

Water and other drinks

Water is something we take for granted. High-quality, fresh water is available from the tap virtually everywhere in the UK. But bottled water is increasingly a drink of choice, while other drinks contain large amounts of water.

Drinking water is generally safe in the UK. Contamination of the water supply is rare, but may cause illness when it occurs. Perhaps the commonest source of contamination is the presence of bacteria from animal faeces. These bacteria do not multiply in water, and are usually not dangerous, but can cause mild gastroenteritis. They are easily killed by boiling, but there should be no bacteria in the water supply. It is simple and cheap to have a sample of water analysed and water authorities have the facilities to do so.

Chemical contamination of water supplies occurs occasionally, usually at such low levels that it is undetectable to consumers, and does not lead to immediate health problems. Problems with water purity seldom occur at its source, although accidents do happen. A large-scale contamination of a water supply with aluminium (safe in tiny amounts and normally used to clear cloudiness from water) occurred in 1988. There are strict regulations about what can be put into water supplies by the providers.

As well as aluminium, chlorine is routinely added to suppress bacteria which might find their way into the supply near to the home.

If you dislike the taste of chlorine in your water, the old-fashioned but still effective remedy is to keep the water in a (covered) jug in the fridge to allow the chlorine to evaporate. Overnight is usually long enough.

If any abnormality is found in your tap water on testing, it is a good idea to check any tanks, and to check the water at the point it enters the house. Normally, cold water taps are supplied directly from the mains pipe, but private water supplies may use header tanks. It can be very difficult to eradicate bacterial contamination of private water supplies. Ultraviolet light treatment is a cheap and reliable solution for domestic supplies.

Always on tap
Tap water quality in the UK is high, and blind tests have revealed that many consumers choose chilled tap water in preference to mineral waters. Water for drinking should always be chosen from a tap supplied directly from the mains.

A quarter of the world's population do not have access to safe drinking water.

BOTTLED OR TAP?
Bottled waters can make a pleasant change and encourage people to drink more. They do have very slightly different tastes, so if you don't like one it is worth trying others. The various health claims made for bottled 'mineral' waters are not, however, founded on evidence. The fizz in almost all 'fizzy' waters – and all of those produced in the UK – is simply added carbon dioxide. It has no relevance to health and can alter the chemical composition of the water. Some waters have this added at the source; others elsewhere.

Water is a natural source of fluoride. In areas of low natural fluoridation, one part per million may be added to the water supply.

The minerals in mineral water

The bottled waters available around the world may contain the following minerals in amounts that vary from traces (in the case of lithium, for example) to more than 1000mg/litre (sodium and potassium). Chemical symbols are given to help you evaluate the mineral content of your favourite water:

- Arsenic (As) • Boron dioxide (BO_2)
- Bromine (Br) • Calcium (Ca)
- Chloride (Cl)
- Carbon dioxide (CO_2)
- Chromium (Cr) • Cobalt (Co)
- Copper (Cu) • Fluoride (F)
- Germanium (Ge)
- Hydrogen carbonate (HCO_3)
- Iodine (I) • Iron (Fe) • Lithium (Li)
- Magnesium (Mg) • Manganese (Mn)
- Nitrate (NO_3) • Potassium (K)
- Rubidium (Rb) • Silica (SiO_2)
- Sodium (Na) • Strontium (Sr)
- Sulphate (SO_4) • Zinc (Zn)

Historically in the UK we have not drunk as much bottled water as in other countries, mainly because our water supplies were of such a high quality. There are almost 500 brands of bottled water in Italy, for example, and nearly 200 in France. This lack of competition from bottled waters has contributed to the huge market for carbonated and sugary drinks in the UK. Without competition from water, these products have become popular, which has had a serious impact on dental health. Few contain fluoride, an essential element for dental health.

The rapid increase in consumption of bottled and canned drinks, especially by younger people, is an interesting phenomenon. Most people would benefit from greater water intake and these drinks should be contributing to this increase: most are around 65 per cent water. But we are not in fact better hydrated for drinking this amount. It may be that we are also consuming so much salt in processed foods that the good effects of extra drinking are being cancelled out.

Types of bottled water

There are essentially two types of bottled water: mineral water and spring water. Spring water, by law, must be collected and bottled at the spring from which it arises. It must meet stringent hygiene standards, but can be treated to remove any impurities and pollutants.

Before emerging from the ground, mineral water naturally picks up various minerals, before it is bottled. Mineral water can only be treated to remove dirt. Since 1999, it has been compulsory in the UK for bottlers to include the mineral content of all waters on the label.

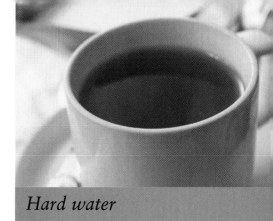

Hard water

Hard water contains dissolved salts of calcium and magnesium. It produces a white crust in kettles, furs up pipes, and needs a lot of soap to make a lather. It is usually viewed as a problem. Water softening units reduce plumbing problems, but they are probably not good for health, and spoil the taste of the water (by adding sodium in exchange for calcium). On the plus side, hard water is rich in calcium, it tastes good, makes the best tea, and there is evidence that people who use hard water have less heart disease.

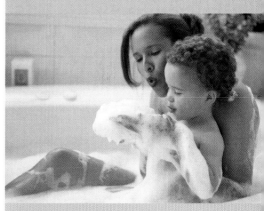

Soft water

Soft water contains little or no dissolved salts of magnesium and calcium. It is kinder to plumbing, makes personal washing and clothes washing easier, it uses less soap and does not leave a 'scum' in the bath. It is by no means a ticket to the coronary care unit, although areas of the UK with high rates of heart disease tend to have soft water. Soft water is without doubt the best to drink with whisky.

How to drink more water

Experts recommend that adults should drink 8–10 250ml glasses of water a day to replace the fluid they lose through sweating, breathing and the digestive process. Anybody who is very active should drink more. Although the body does absorb some water from food, nutritionists recommend only counting fluid from drinks in your daily total. Here are some ideas for getting more water into your daily routine.

1 Drink regularly

If you drink little and often, you are not going to overload the kidneys – which will in any case simply get rid of what your body doesn't need – or your bladder. Drinking small amounts regularly keeps the whole body hydrated.

2 Water on the move

Carry a bottle of water with you when out walking or on public transport, and have a bottle in a cool bag in the car. Sip from it frequently so that you don't become dehydrated while out and about. This is especially important in warm weather – remember you are still losing fluid even if you aren't sweating.

In 2001, 1600 million litres of mineral water were sold in the UK, at a value of £900 million. The French drink four times this amount.

3 Water at your desk

If there is a water cooler in your workplace, visit it regularly. Otherwise, keep a bottle of water on your desk and drink from it at least every half an hour. The warm, dry air in many buildings – including offices, schools and hospitals – is especially dehydrating.

4 Be wise to social diuretics

Tea, coffee and alcoholic drinks all have a social value, but all generate extra urine. These drinks demand water: always drink a glass of water at the same time.

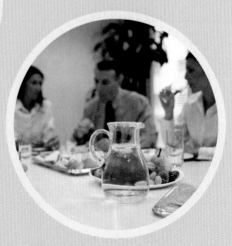

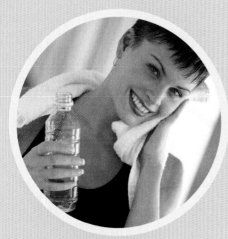

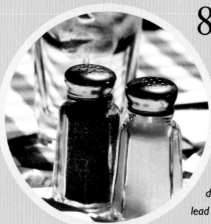

8 Reduce salt intake

Salt causes the body to retain water, and the more salt you contain, the more water you need to flush through the kidneys. It is better for you and your kidneys to avoid this double overload by reducing the amount of salt you eat. Adding a little salt at the table to fresh, whole foods cooked without salt should not pose risks to health, but a diet high in processed foods is likely to lead to significantly more salt being eaten than you are aware of and is good for health.

9 At the gym

You need at least a glass of water for every 30 minutes exercise you take, so take a sports bottle with you. Drink water after a swim – even though you have been in water, the exercise will contribute to dehydration.

7 Before a meal

Drink a glass of water before a meal, especially if you are trying to control your weight. This will make you feel fuller, so you eat less – and water has no calories. This is especially important if you will be drinking alcohol or coffee with your meal.

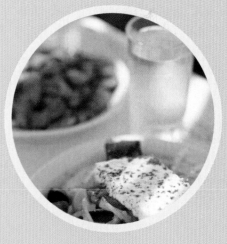

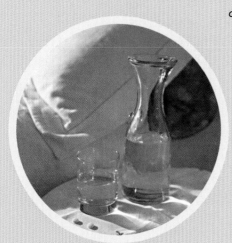

6 Flavour to go

Many bottled waters now come in interesting flavours and colours, some more natural than others. It's best to read the labels on these: some contain sugar or artificial sweeteners. If you don't like the taste of your tap water, consider fitting a filter or use a filter jug (but change the filter regularly). If you can't find a plain bottled water you like, try a fruit-flavoured infusion – these are naturally caffeine free.

5 Rise and shine

Have a glass of water first thing in the morning, before you have your breakfast. This could be warm if you prefer. Try adding a slice of lemon or lime to wake up your palate. During the winter you could also add a vitamin C tablet.

WHAT ELSE CONTAINS WATER?

In the UK the major sources of water include tea and coffee, and also beer and wine, for those who drink them. All these drinks are mostly water, but they all have both positive and negative effects on health. Tea contributes a daily average of 253ml of water to the diet, coffee 312ml and carbonated drinks 266ml. The average daily consumption of water from alcohol is very low on account of the large number of people who do not drink alcohol at all.

All of these drinks are pure from a microbiological point of view, that is they contain no harmful bugs, but all may contain traces of residues of pesticides and herbicides. In some countries – though generally not in Europe – the regulations governing growing conditions are very lax.

We consume more than 5500 million litres of carbonated soft drinks every year in the UK, that's 100 litres per person.

All also have a diuretic effect, that is they increase the production of urine. Of course the normal physiological diuretic is water itself. Drinking diuretics triggers a complex series of hormones to relay a message to the kidneys (and to sweat glands) to produce more dilute, watery, urine.

Other diuretics, including caffeine, alcohol and diuretic tablets, interfere with this control of fluid balance to produce more dilute urine – that is, they lose more water than is stimulated by the water intake alone.

Thus these drinks, if consumed as the only source of water, would lead to mild dehydration and a variety of symptoms. The answer is to cover their consumption with extra water.

Fruit juices and drinks

Pure fruit and vegetable juices are 90 per cent water, so as well as contributing to the recommended daily intake of five portions of fruit and vegetables for health, they will also help to keep you hydrated. Fruit juices contain the same vitamins and minerals as fresh fruit, but do not contain the fibre.

Fruit juice drinks and squashes, although they contribute to water intake, do not have the same health benefits as pure juice and may contain sugar and other additives. It is kinder to teeth if sugary drinks are only taken with food.

How healthy is your tipple?

		Positive	Negative
	WATER	Free and delicious. The best solution to and preventer of dehydration.	Contamination, particularly in rural areas where private supplies may require sterilisation.
	FRUIT JUICE	Pure juice contains vitamins and minerals; a major source of vitamin C and folic acid.	Acidity of fruit sugars can damage teeth.
	TEA AND COFFEE	Contain caffeine which stimulates the brain and improves respiratory function. Potassium replaces body cells. Antioxidant phenolic compounds in tea (but not coffee) protect against free radical damage.	Caffeine can cause palpitations, anxiety and insomnia and is a diuretic. Phenolic compounds and others in tea may block iron absorption and cause constipation.
	WINE AND BEER	Alcoholic drinks have social and symbolic importance. Antioxidant phenolic compounds in red wine protect against free radical damage.	Alcohol can intoxicate and is a diuretic. Alcohol also weakens the willpower with respect to dieting.
	SWEETENED FIZZY DRINKS	Caffeine in cola drinks may stimulate brain and respiratory function.	Caffeine (as coffee). Acid dissolves tooth enamel. High sugar content leads to tooth decay.

Dehydration

Many people would feel better if they drank more water, and many common day-to-day symptoms are aggravated by not drinking enough. In certain circumstances drinking more water is vital if we are to avoid ill health.

As a land species our relationship with water is always critical, and we are vulnerable to the imbalance which leads to mild dehydration. Unchecked dehydration can mean death, so we have sophisticated systems to conserve and retain water. Our skin keeps the inside in and the outside out, but originally the skin's main function, complemented by the kidneys, was to stop us becoming diluted in a watery environment.

Rejuvenating fluid
Water helps to keep the skin well hydrated, which makes it stay younger looking. It also feels softer to the touch. Adequate hydration is good for all body systems, however.

THE HEALTH BENEFITS OF GOOD HYDRATION

Being well hydrated has notable benefits for the bladder and urinary tract. It makes infections less likely (see page 48) and some studies have shown that good hydration can decrease the risk of kidney stones. There are health benefits for almost every body system.

- The eyes and skin remain moist and healthy: skin looks younger and eyes feel less 'gritty'.
- The digestive system works more efficiently, making constipation less likely and stools easier to pass.
- Both mental and physical endurance are improved.
- The mood is lifted: dehydration tends to make people irritable and short tempered.
- The muscles and joints work smoothly and freely, avoiding stiffness or cramps.
  - Headaches and migraines become less common.

A timely drink of water may fend off a threatened headache.
- Breastfeeding mothers have fewer problems with milk production if they are drinking enough themselves.
- Good hydration improves lung function. It may help asthmatics to avoid attacks, and avoids the accumulation of congealed secretions in the airways.

positive health tips

Hydration in the home

Modern central heating and electric heating provide hot dry air – unlike open fires or gas fires, which release water vapour into the air. This contributes to the body's water loss indoors, which is greater than outdoors. This applies particularly at night and at work, and in schools and hospitals. A number of troublesome symptoms like headaches and difficulty concentrating can result from this mild dehydration. Possible counter-measures include:

- Set saucers of water on radiators – or buy a humidifier. These will add water vapour to the air and reduce water loss, but at the additional cost of causing condensation (with the possibility of fungal growth generating spores which can cause respiratory problems).

- A better solution is simply to drink more. You could also keep the windows open more often and compensate by wearing an extra layer of clothing.

WHAT IS DEHYDRATION?

Dehydration occurs when the body loses more fluid than it takes in. This can happen in obvious situations – during hard manual work or exercise in hot weather, for example. But it can also occur in many other situations. It is especially common in the elderly, the ill and the immobile.

The warning signs of even mild dehydration are usually obvious but often overlooked. They include a dry mouth and throat. Even low levels of fluid loss can affect concentration and energy levels. Severe dehydration is a medical emergency and may need hospitalisation and intravenous fluids to restore fluid levels. People die from dehydration.

Warning signs of dehydration

These include:
• dizziness or lightheadedness;
• thirst;
• headache;
• nausea;
• tiredness;
• loss of appetite.
Babies and small children may also be lethargic. In a baby, the eyes and fontanelle may be sunken.

WATER AND SPORTS

Physical activity generates metabolic products, which need to be removed from the body. Respiration increases during exercise, and so water loss is increased by evaporation in the breath as well as by perspiration.

The water losses during sporting activities can be measured by weight change, which generally shows a rate of loss of about a litre an hour – more at higher temperatures and with exceptional exertion. Sporting performance is affected by very minor degrees of dehydration of the order of 2 per cent, so extra water is needed for any competitive sport which lasts more than 30 minutes.

It is important to start with good hydration, and useful to have some water already available in the gut (although not too much in the stomach). Drinking 400–500ml half an hour before starting to exercise is sensible, as is drinking at a similar rate while training. Check your urine colour before you start your session: it should be pale or even colourless.

During exercise itself, water is better absorbed by the body if it contains 3–5 per cent glucose and a

A dehydration rate of 4 per cent causes a 22 per cent decrease in sporting performance.

little sodium. This is one good reason to drink glucose-electrolyte sports drinks. The amount of energy (as glucose) has no value except in very prolonged activity, such as marathon running for example. After training, and after sports events, check your urine colour again. If you have drunk enough it will still be pale.

HYDRATION AND HOLIDAYS

It can be more difficult to maintain good hydration in unfamiliar surroundings or when out of the normal routine. Staying hydrated, however, need not be tricky if you know when extra liquid is needed.

Water and altitude

The loss of water through breath increases when breathing is more rapid, when the air is dry, and at low atmospheric pressure – all these conditions apply at altitude. Mountaineers above about 1000m (3300ft), for example, need more water than usual, and more than for the same exertion at sea level.

Water and flying

Aircraft are customarily pressurised to reduce the effect of altitude, but the pressure is equivalent to walking at a height of 2000–3000m (6600–9900ft), and the air is very dry. For these reasons dehydration is common during long flights, and is aggravated by alcohol and caffeine. Prolonged waiting in airports

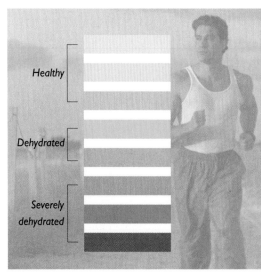

Healthy

Dehydrated

Severely dehydrated

AM I DEHYDRATED?

It's not necessary to drink constantly, but it is important to maintain a regular water intake throughout the day of at least 1.5–2 litres. A simple way to check if you have drunk enough is to check the colour of your urine. The paler the urine is, the better: dark urine could indicate dehydration.

without access to drinking water makes things worse. One of the serious complications of dehydration – venous thrombosis and other emboli – is further provoked by inactivity and a cramped position. This condition can be fatal. Maintaining higher than normal water consumption on long flights is therefore vital. As a guide, 500ml is needed for each 1000km (625 miles). Therefore on a transatlantic flight you should aim to drink about 2 litres of water – more if you also drink coffee, tea, cola or alcohol.

Avoiding traveller's tummy

Part of the key to avoiding traveller's tummy is to arrive hydrated and start to drink more if the weather is warm and the atmosphere dry, or if you are doing anything strenuous.

Traveller's diarrhoea usually comes from contaminated food, rather than contaminated water, but it is worth taking sensible precautions.

- If you are not sure of the local drinking water, drink bottled water from bottles with intact seals when you buy them, or boil water for drinking, ice-making and tooth-brushing for 10 minutes before use.
- Avoid ice cubes in drinks as these will probably have been made with tap water.
- Peel all fruit and vegetables or wash them in bottled water.

- Avoid pre-cooked meat products. Some experts recommend eating only local dishes as chefs are more practised in their handling and storage.
- Do not eat mayonnaise or ice creams from machines; they may not have been stored constantly at optimal temperatures.
- Don't 'rehydrate' with alcohol: this causes the kidneys to produce more urine, increasing dehydration.

If despite your precautions, you are ill, take an oral electrolyte solution. These may be available over the counter in some areas. Otherwise, mix a quarter of a teaspoon of salt and 3 level teaspoons of sugar in 600ml boiled water.

WATER AND ILLNESS

High water loss from vomiting or diarrhoea, and reduced intake through nausea or immobility, are common symptoms of many different illnesses. At the same time, water loss through the breath and skin are increased by fever. Dehydration is therefore a frequent feature of illness. It is a particular problem in infants and in the elderly, since in addition to the symptoms of dehydration, it results in a high risk of kidney failure.

Increased water consumption, often to levels above those that an ill person may feel like drinking, is therefore necessary in illness. Intravenous or subcutaneous fluids can be given to very sick people or those who are severely dehydrated, but even if a person is vomiting, continuing to drink frequently, in modest amounts, encourages absorption of some water – not all will be vomited away.

A fast pulse, and falling blood pressure, is a sign of dehydration.

KEEPING KIDS HYDRATED

Children are at greater risk of dehydration at all ages than adults. Babies and infants are more prone to vomiting and diarrhoea and more vulnerable to their effects, tolerating the loss of fluid less well than adults who have a greater overall body weight. Young children run around more than adults do, and tend not to notice that they are thirsty, or ignore their thirst while they are playing. Toddlers may not be able to tell you that they are thirsty. They are also likely to be outdoors during the warmer hours of the day.

American studies suggest that most children only drink half as much water as they should. Schoolchildren may spend hours at a time in warm classrooms with little access to drinking water. Although the effect of adequate hydration on brain function is being increasingly acknowledged, many schools still do not encourage children to drink water regularly throughout the day.

To ensure that your children are drinking enough water:

- Set a good example, by drinking plenty of water yourself.
- Limit the alternatives to water: a child who is not offered sugary drinks or fruit juice will be happy with the taste of water.
- Add slices of fresh fruit to water, or make 'cocktails': juice some interesting fruit like a kiwi fruit or some strawberries and serve topped up half and half with sparkling mineral water.
- Use fun cups and interestingly shaped straws, or sports bottles, so that drinking becomes associated with playing.
- Make ice cubes from water with a touch of fruit juice added, in lots of interesting shapes, so that water is always cool.
- Make ice lollies from diluted fruit juices for children to suck.
- Work with your child's school to improve children's access to water – this may mean taking a sports bottle in to school each day and active encouragement by staff to drink regularly during lessons and breaks.

Fruit and star burst
Ice cubes made with a little added fruit juice, or even frozen around a piece of fresh fruit, will liven up a glass of water for a child (above). Or freeze water and juice mixes to serve as ice lollies and sorbets (below).

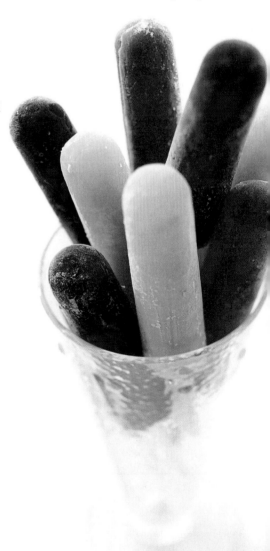

EATING FOR KIDNEY HEALTH

The food and drink we consume has a major impact on health in general, but nowhere is this more apparent than the kidneys and bladder. Overloading the system with substances that the kidneys recognise as poisons, or that irritate the urinary system, can lead to ill health: kidney-friendly foods, by contrast, can boost well-being.

 74 Eating well is vital for overall health, but it pays extra dividends for the kidneys and bladder if you have a generally healthy diet.

 75 Many of us eat far more protein each day than is recommended, which has an impact on the kidneys' workload.

 77 Medical thinking has changed with regard to calcium and the kidneys, and doctors now believe that limiting calcium intake is unwise.

 78 Salt intake can have a major impact on kidney health: here are tips on how to cut down, without compromising on flavour.

 82 Increasing your intake of friendly bacteria can go a long way toward improving the health of your urinary system: find out how and why.

Eat a protective, nutrient-dense diet

Help keep your kidneys and urinary tract healthy by eating foods that reduce high blood pressure, keep kidney stones at bay and combat other diseases and disorders that can affect the urinary system.

A diet that is good for your kidneys is a good, basic, nutritionally sound eating plan that will not put any undue strain on your kidneys or aggravate any existing kidney or urinary tract condition.

EATING TO MAINTAIN HEALTHY KIDNEYS

Try to eat a varied range of foods each day. Aim for an assortment of animal and vegetable proteins, and balance the rest of your diet by including high-fibre and low-fat foods such as wholegrain cereals.

To ensure overall health, it's best to choose reduced fat dairy products and meat cuts whenever you can, and to meet the five-portions-a-day target for fruit and vegetables.

Your diet should include:
- high-fibre foods
- low-fat foods
- plenty of fruit and vegetables
- wholegrain breads and cereals
- beans, peas and other pulses
- low-fat dairy products
- small amounts of lean meat, fish and chicken, to reduce the burden of work that a high-protein diet imposes on the kidneys.

BE WISE IF THERE'S A PROBLEM

People with a kidney disorder or disease may need to follow a low-protein diet to prevent further damage to their kidneys. They may also have to restrict their intake of sodium and potassium-rich foods.

If you have a urinary tract infection, avoid foods and drinks that irritate the bladder. This often includes caffeine, spicy foods and alcohol.

A healthy day

A healthy body makes for healthy kidneys, so all good general nutrition rules apply. A sample healthy day's menu might look like this:

BREAKFAST
1 medium-sized bowl of muesli with a handful of fresh strawberries served with 250ml semi-skimmed milk
1 thick slice of wholegrain bread with low-fat spread
1 glass of apple juice

LUNCH
1 medium-sized baked potato with 2 tablespoons of baked beans (containing reduced salt and reduced sugar)
1 large serving of green salad with fat-free dressing
A handful of grapes
1 pot of low-fat yogurt

DINNER
1 lean lamb chop, grilled and served with mixed vegetables
1 bowl of brown rice salad
1 baked apple with raisins

SNACKS
Fruit, breadsticks, rye crackers, low-fat cheese

Don't forget breakfast!
Studies have shown that a bowl of wholegrain cereal every morning can help to lower blood pressure, and therefore reduce the risk of kidney failure. You could try mixing different grains and add fresh fruit for a nutritious start to the day.

Protein and your kidneys

Protein is vital for the body's growth and repair. Too much protein is not good for the kidneys, however – nor is too little. Keep your kidneys happy by taking in a sensible mix of animal and plant proteins, in moderate amounts.

DAILY PROTEIN NEEDS

Protein is constantly being broken down into amino acids to make new tissues in the body. The daily protein requirement of a healthy adult eating a mixed diet is 0.75g of protein per kilogram of body weight. This means that an adult weighing 60kg (9st 6lb) requires 45g (1½oz) of protein a day.

Our daily protein requirements are best fulfilled by eating a diet that includes a mix of animal and vegetable proteins to ensure that we meet our basic amino acid requirements. Animal proteins provided by meat, fish, eggs, milk and cheese have high proportions of indispensable (essential) amino acids. Indispensable amino acids can't be made in the body in amounts large enough to keep us healthy, and so must be provided by our food.

Vegetable proteins found in nuts, seeds, pulses and cereals have low levels of indispensable amino acids.

What if protein intake is lower than recommended levels?

In healthy adults the total amount of protein in the body can vary widely without having a serious effect on health, so long as enough energy-giving calories are being eaten as well. If this is not the case, protein will be broken down to meet the body's energy requirements instead.

Therefore, over a period of time protein deficiency can develop from either a very low protein intake or a

Sources of protein

Many foods contain a high concentration of protein, so even a small quantity can fulfil your daily protein requirements. Nuts in particular are an excellent source of protein.

FOOD	SERVING SIZE	GRAMS (g) OF PROTEIN
Cheddar cheese	40g (1 chunk)	10.2
Lamb chump chop, grilled	70g (1 chop)	19.6
Pork loin chop, grilled	75g (1 chop)	31.4
Sirloin steak, grilled	110g (1 steak)	29.0
Pork sausage, grilled	40g (1 large)	5.8
Chicken drumstick, roasted	90g (1)	23.9
Turkey breast, roasted	70g (3 slices)	20.2
Trout, grilled	115g (1 whole trout)	33.3
Prawns, boiled	60g (20 peeled prawns)	13.6
Baked beans	80g (portion)	3.8
White bread	36g (1 slice)	3.0
Potato, baked	100g (1 small)	3.8
Quorn	70g (1 portion)	8.3
Peanuts	13g (10 peanuts)	3.0
Sesame seeds	12g (1 tablespoon)	2.0
Lentils, boiled	80g (2 tablespoons)	7.0
Tofu, steamed	60g (1 portion)	4.9
Red kidney beans, boiled	70g (2 tablespoons)	4.8
Milk	125ml	4.1
Egg, boiled	60g (1 egg)	7.5

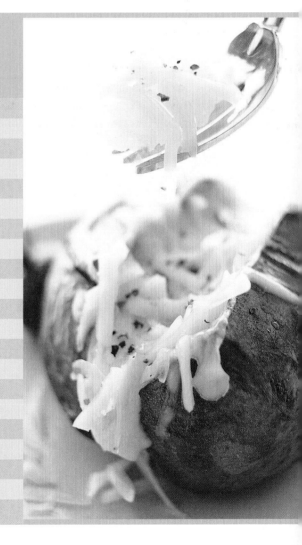

Studies show that some people in the UK consume twice their daily protein requirement.

low calorie intake. Typical symptoms of protein deficiency – known as protein-energy malnutrition – include anaemia, an increased risk of infection, the slow healing of wounds and muscle wasting. Protein-energy malnutrition can occur among people who have anorexia nervosa, AIDS or cancer; it can also be a consequence of old age.

Can you eat too much protein?
In the UK the average adult male eats around 85g of protein a day and a women eats around 62g a day – far more than most people need.

When protein intake is higher than the body requires, a healthy adult's body gets rid of the excess via the kidneys and urinary system. Since excess protein can't be stored, eating a high-protein diet has no health benefits and can put kidneys under pressure.

Protein for kidney health
If you want to lessen the workload of your kidneys, reducing the amount of waste products that they need to excrete makes good sense. Protein metabolism produces

urea. When protein intake is too high this increases the chances of over-stretching the capacity of the kidneys, as they struggle to eliminate urea from the body. This is particularly dangerous for people with diabetes, and those who are already experiencing problems with their kidneys. In addition, high protein intake at the expense of other nutrients can cause bones to lose calcium, and can also raise blood pressure levels.

Animal protein appears to have a more harmful effect on the kidneys than vegetable protein. So it's a good idea to increase the proportion of protein that you eat from plant sources, such as soya.

Researchers' recommendations are that adults should not eat more than 1.5g of protein per kilogram of body weight per day, which works out at a maximum of 90g of protein per day for an adult weighing 60kg.

High protein/ low carbohydrate diets: good or bad for kidneys?

Diets that combine a high protein intake with a low carbohydrate intake – such as the popular Atkins diet – can be dangerous for people with kidney disease, high blood pressure or diabetes. If your carbohydrate intake is low, the body turns instead to stored carbohydrate (glycogen) from the liver and muscles for energy. Once this has been used up, the body uses protein for fuel. A side effect of using protein in this way is the production of acidic compounds called ketones that build up in the blood and urine and can damage the kidneys further, and worsen high blood pressure and diabetic conditions. The risk of heart disease is also greater, due to the increased intake of foods high in fat, particularly saturated fat.

ASK THE EXPERT

Protein for the day
An adult only needs to consume 0.75g of protein per kilo of bodyweight each day. This means that a person weighing 60kg requires just 45g of protein a day – that could be made up by just two chicken drumsticks. But you do not need to get your protein solely from meat, it can come from a range of sources including milk, eggs, cheese and vegetables – all of which contain many vital nutrients.

Calcium and your kidneys

Four out of every five kidney stones are made of calcium oxalate. Can altering the amount of calcium and oxalate that you take in actually reduce the risk of developing calcium-oxalate stones?

Calcium is an important mineral, needed for the formation of strong bones and teeth. A good intake of calcium throughout a person's life will improve their health, and help to prevent osteoporosis.

Oxalate is a substance derived from oxalic acid. It is chiefly found in whole grains, fruit and vegetables. It has no nutritional value in itself, but it can bind to calcium.

Should we limit our calcium intake?

The more calcium-rich foods you eat, the more calcium you produce and the more calcium is excreted via the kidneys. With this in mind, it has been thought that a high calcium intake over-burdens the kidneys, and therefore encourages the production of calcium-oxalate kidney stones.

Recent research, however, has shown that limiting calcium to half the recommended intake of 700mg a day for adults, does not reduce the number of kidney stones. In fact, a study of 45,000 healthy men with no history of kidney stones who were put on high-calcium diets, subsequently developed a third less kidney stones than might have been expected for their sex and age group. It would therefore appear that a high-calcium diet actually lessens the chances of developing kidney stones.

In general, doctors recommend that patients with calcium-oxalate stones do not restrict their calcium intake, so as to avoid osteoporosis.

Should we eat less oxalate?

Since oxalate can bind with calcium to form kidney stones, it would seem logical to eat less oxalate in the hope of reducing the chances of developing a kidney stone.

Sources of oxalate include spinach, beetroot, celery, nuts, rhubarb, strawberries, tea, instant coffee and chocolate. Surprisingly, however, studies have shown that not much more than a tenth of the oxalate present in urine is derived from the food you eat. Therefore it is debatable whether reducing your intake of oxalate lessens the risk of suffering from kidney stones. Nevertheless, most experts agree that those who normally eat a oxalate-rich diet could benefit from eating fewer oxalate-rich foods.

Should we reduce our intake of vitamin D?

Vitamin D plays a vital role in the absorption of calcium. However, the more vitamin D there is circulating in your blood, the more calcium you excrete through your kidneys. Some researchers think that too much vitamin D can encourage kidney stones. So topping up the amount of vitamin D naturally produced in your body, with dietary supplements or by sunbathing, may encourage the formation of calcium-oxalate stones.

However, this area remains controversial and so far there is no evidence to prove this.

SOURCES OF CALCIUM	
FOOD	MG CALCIUM PER SERVING
125ml Milk	150
125ml Yoghurt	188
40g Cheddar cheese	324
50g Canned sardines with bones	275
36g White bread	40
36g Wholemeal bread	19
20g Watercress	34
90g Spinach	144
30g Sultanas	19
50g Boiled okra	60

Reduce salt intake

Cutting back on salt will help to reduce high blood pressure – a key strategy when maintaining kidney health. In a two-way link, high blood pressure may cause kidney damage, and poor kidney function can cause high blood pressure.

High blood pressure – also known as hypertension – is a major cause of coronary heart disease and strokes, especially in people who have diabetes as well.

The link between salt and hypertension

Research has shown a link between high sodium intake (mostly in the form of salt) and high blood pressure, especially among people who are older. Some say, however, that the link is not strong enough to indicate for certain whether healthy younger adults with normal blood pressure need to reduce their sodium intake. Certainly, if you are older, or have high blood pressure, it is worth cutting down on your sodium intake. But you might want to keep in mind that carrying too much weight and drinking too much alcohol both have a much greater effect on raising your blood pressure level.

How much sodium do we need?

The body needs between 0.07g and 0.4g of sodium a day to stay healthy. The average sodium intake per person in the UK is about ten times that amount – around 3.9g per day, equal to 9g of salt. Most of this comes from processed foods. Doctors recommend that adults aim to eat no more than 1.6g of sodium per day, equal to 6g of salt (6000mg), which is a realistic amount to achieve, and should have a measurable effect on high blood pressure.

Sources of sodium in food

Sodium and chloride levels are fairly low in any foods that have not been processed. Extra salt is added to many prepared foods, however, so that meat (especially pork) and fish which are not high in salt in their natural state become rich sources of salt if eaten as ham, sausages, bacon or kippers. Salt is also added to

SODIUM IN THE DIET

Some quite unexpected foods can be sources of sodium. Anyone who is looking to limit salt intake should know that most food labels quote a product's sodium levels. To work out the equivalent in grams of salt, multiply the sodium value by 2.5.

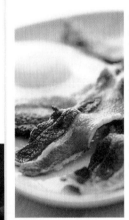

Some meat products can be high in salt. Topping the list is corned beef: a thick slice (50g) contains more than a gram of salt. A rasher of streaky bacon and an average pork sausage both contain 750mg of salt.

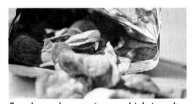

Snacks and savouries are high in salt. A standard (30g) bag of potato crisps contains 803 milligrams of salt. A teaspoon (5g) of Marmite will add 563mg of salt to your daily total, while the same amount of soy sauce adds 715mg.

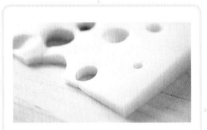

Dairy products are moderate sources of salt. A chunk (45g) of Cheddar cheese contains 755mg of salt, while 250ml (½ pint) of milk adds 402mg to the diet. Salted butter and margarine both contain 10mg of salt per 5g serving.

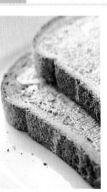

Bread can be a rich source of salt. An average slice from a large loaf (about 36g) contains 187mg sodium, equivalent to 468mg of salt.

butter (unless unsalted), margarine, canned vegetables, canned meat, bread, snacks, breakfast cereals, cheese, condiments such as mustard, marinades and many other products. In addition, sodium goes into monosodium glutamate and sodium bicarbonate (baking powder).

Eating less salt

Most of us eat more salt than we need. There is no evidence to suggest that a reduction might be harmful, and it may help, so it's worth making an effort to cut down on your intake. Here are some tips to help you reduce the amount of salt you eat.
- Choose fresh foods.
- Avoid processed and packaged foods.
- Don't add salt to food at the table.
- Don't add salt to the water when boiling vegetables.
- Try to add less salt when cooking in general.
- Be sure to eat your five daily servings of fruits and vegetables (naturally low in sodium).
- Cut down on convenience meals, snacks, pickles and smoked foods.
- Use low-sodium baking powder, snacks, pickles and smoked foods.
- Buy unsalted butter.

Potassium and your kidneys

Our bodies need potassium for a variety of reasons. Potassium and sodium work together to regulate water retention and blood pressure. Potassium is chiefly found in fruit, and also in vegetables, beans and milk. The kidneys help to maintain just the right amount of potassium in the blood by excreting the excess in urine. Most people can absorb up to 18g of potassium a day. In fact, potassium toxicity – a condition called hyperkalemia – is very unlikely to occur unless you take potassium supplements inappropriately. If you have problems with your kidneys, potassium retention may become a concern, and could result in heart failure. Therefore, the doctor may advise you to restrict your intake of potassium-rich foods.

On the other hand, if you are prone to developing kidney stones it is desirable to keep potassium levels high. This is because potassium citrate in combination with magnesium citrate appears to help deter kidney stones from forming. Potassium levels are best boosted by eating fruit and vegetables, in which there is much more potassium than in supplements. Another drawback of supplements is that they can irritate the stomach.

Will soya products affect my kidneys?

Processed soya products are all high in sodium and so should be avoided, along with other foods containing sodium, if you already have high blood pressure.
There are more processed food products made from soya beans than you might imagine. They include textured vegetable protein (TVP), tofu, miso, soy sauce, soya milk, soya oil and soya margarine. As with all nutritional foods containing sodium, however, there is no reason to avoid eating soya products if your blood pressure is within normal levels. Indeed, soya protein is easier on the kidneys than animal protein. Unprocessed soya beans do not raise blood pressure levels and can be safely included in any healthy diet.

ASK THE EXPERT

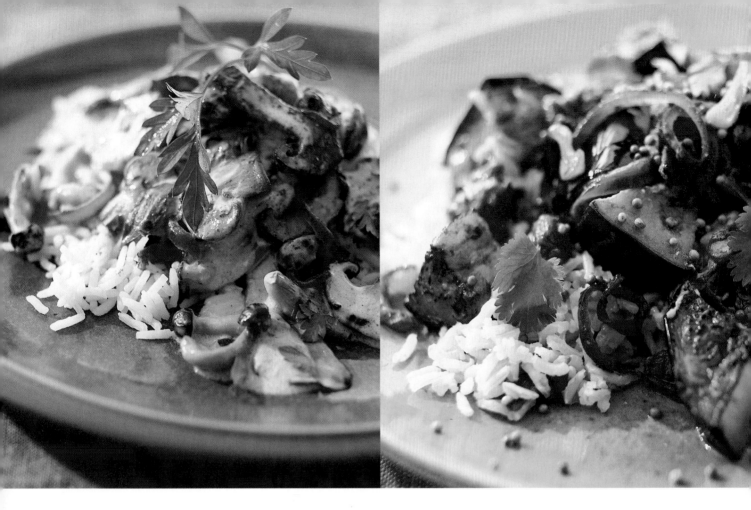

LOW-SALT RECIPES

Most people have grown used to eating salty flavours, usually to the detriment of more subtle ones. It is, however, possible to prepare tasty meals without relying on salt. People who use less salt when cooking find that the true flavours of foods start to come through.

Ways of adding flavour to foods without using salt

- Sprinkle vegetables with herbs, spices, lime or lemon juice instead of using salt.
- Use spices such as coriander, cumin and pepper.
- Use lemon juice or olive oil flavoured with herbs, to marinade meat and vegetables.
- Use gomasio (a mix of toasted, crushed sesame seeds and salt).
- Use low-sodium salt, and low-salt versions of fermented sauces, such as tamari, shoyu or miso.

MUSHROOM STROGANOFF

1 tbsp olive oil
1 large onion, chopped
1kg mixed mushrooms (such as button, chestnut and shiitaki), sliced
½ tsp Dijon mustard
200ml low-fat crème fraîche
pinch fresh nutmeg
pinch paprika
chopped flat-leaf parsley

Heat the oil in a pan, and fry the onion until translucent (10–15 minutes over medium heat). Add the sliced mushrooms, and fry for another 5–7 minutes. Add the Dijon mustard and crème fraîche, stir and then add the nutmeg and paprika. Add the parsley before serving with plain boiled white rice.
Serves 4.

AUBERGINE CURRY

2 tbsp olive oil
1 tsp mustard seeds
1 large onion, chopped
2 cloves of garlic, crushed
1 tbsp grated ginger
1 tsp turmeric
1 tsp cayenne pepper
1 tsp ground cumin
2 tbsp cornflour
3 large aubergines, cut into cubes
1 large can chopped tomatoes
pinch of low-sodium salt (optional)
1 pot low fat yoghurt
a handful of chopped coriander

Heat the oil in a pan, fry the mustard seeds until they start to pop, then add the onion, garlic and ginger, fry for 10–15 minutes on low heat until the onions have turned translucent. Add the spices, sprinkle in the cornflour and stir. Turn up the heat, add the aubergine cubes and stir fry for about 5 minutes.

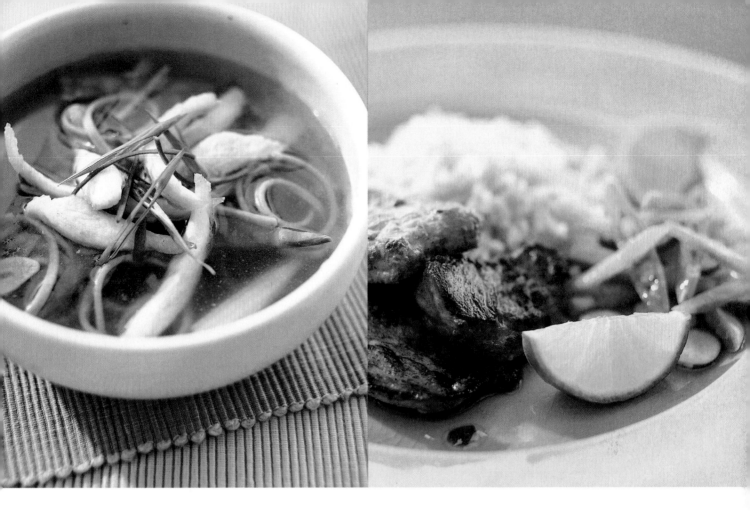

Add the canned tomatoes, allow to boil, then turn the heat down. Cover and simmer for 10–15 minutes or until the aubergines are soft. Season with low-sodium salt if desired, mix in the yoghurt and chopped coriander and serve with boiled white rice.
Serves 4.

CHICKEN AND NOODLES IN A FRAGRANT THAI BROTH

60g dried wholewheat noodles
450ml homemade chicken stock
1 red chilli, deseeded and chopped
1 clove garlic, crushed
2 tsp finely shredded ginger
2 tsp shoyu sauce
50g mangetout
50g baby sweetcorn
1 tbsp sunflower oil
175g chicken breast cut into strips
lime juice
a handful of basil leaves

Cook the noodles, according to instructions on the packet, rinse under cold water and drain. Bring the chicken stock to the boil with the chilli, garlic, ginger and shoyu sauce to the boil. Add the vegetables and boil for 5 minutes. Meanwhile, heat the oil in a pan, stir fry the chicken strips for 5–7 minutes or until cooked. Assemble the dish by placing the noodles in a large bowl, pour over the stock with the cooked vegetables. Place the cooked chicken strips on top, and add a sprinkling of lime juice. Sprinkle with basil leaves just before serving.
If you wish serve with extra lime juice, fresh beansprouts and chopped coriander.
Serves 4.

PORK SUKIYAKI
Marinade:
2 tbsp tamari sauce
570ml water
3 large shallots, minced
1 large clove garlic, crushed
1 tsp freshly grated ginger
1 tbsp white wine vinegar
1 tbsp honey
1 tsp sesame oil
450g lean pork, such as fillet, sliced
vegetable oil for frying.

Combine the marinade ingredients in a bowl, add the pork and leave to marinade for 10–15 minutes. Remove the pork from the marinade. Heat the oil in a pan, add the pork slices and fry for 3 minutes on each side or until cooked. Serve with boiled brown rice and salad vegetables such as grated carrots, celery and mooli, dressed with oil and lime juice vinaigrette.
Serves 4.

Boost your intake of lactobacilli

Lactobacilli – lactic acid bacteria – have important health giving properties. By combating infection in the gut and boosting the immune system in general, they help to keep infection at bay within the kidneys and urinary tract.

What are lactobacilli?

Lactobacilli are lactic acid bacteria that are added to pasteurised milk to break down the sugar found in milk (called lactose) into lactic acid and turn the milk into yoghurt.

They are also used when making cheese, sour milk and fermented yoghurt drinks.

Lactobacilli for a healthy body

Lactobacilli are 'friendly' bacteria that increase the acidity level in the gut. This inhibits the growth of potentially harmful micro-organisms and as a result encourages desirable bacteria to flourish instead.

This helps the immune system to function more effectively and so fight off infection more successfully. This is of particular benefit to anyone with a urinary tract infection.

People with yeast infections – usually caused by the fungus Candida albicans – have found that consuming foods containing lactobacilli helps to reduce their symptoms.

To guarantee an intake of helpful bacteria you could try bio-yoghurts or probiotic dietary supplements, which contain

bacteria such as Acidophilus, Bifidus and Bugaricus. The only difference is that the bacteria in the yoghurt are live, while the bacteria in the supplements have been freeze-dried. This means they are in a dormant state until re-hydrated in the gut.

Yoghurt culture

Brands of yoghurt vary greatly in the strain of bacteria they contain and some do not contain any live bacteria. Bio-yoghurts have high levels of friendly bacteria.

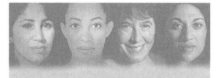

A DIET TO COMBAT YEAST INFECTIONS

If you suspect you have a yeast infection, it's important to consult your GP for advice on treatment, but in addition to any treatment prescribed by your doctor, a special diet may also be of benefit. Such a diet can be pretty severe, however, so don't embark on one without consulting your doctor; together, you can work out a balanced eating plan that will cover all your nutritional needs.

Diets designed to combat Candida and other yeast infections suggest that you avoid all yeast-containing foods (such as bread and yeast extracts), sugar and artificial sweeteners, refined grains (white flour, white rice, white pasta), fermented products (soy sauce, vinegar, ketchup), cow's milk, fresh and dried fruits, nuts, smoked and fermented meats and fish (such as ham, smoked fish), tea and coffee, mushrooms and spices.

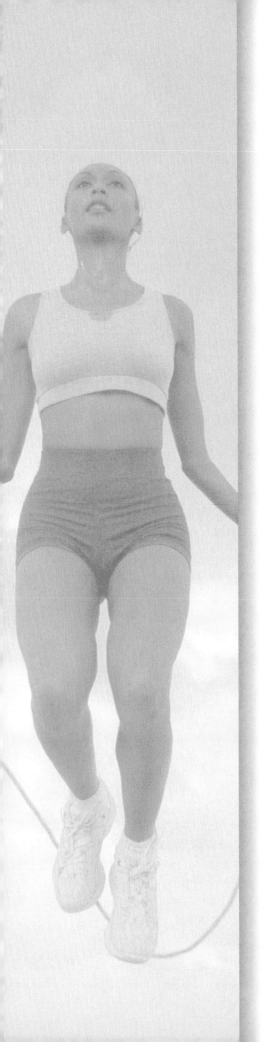

EXERCISE AND THE KIDNEYS

Exercise keeps the kidneys healthy, improving blood flow through them and preserving the body's core temperature. Exercise can also improve bladder health, since keeping muscles toned can help to prevent incontinence. But exercise is not only for the fit; people who have kidney problems can improve their fitness level with a tailored programme.

84 *Exercise has enormous benefits for kidney and urinary health, especially if some sensible precautions are taken.*

87 *Research has shown that people with kidney problems can improve their symptoms and quality of life through exercise.*

88 *Pelvic floor exercises are crucial to health: they can help to prevent the embarrassing, troublesome condition of stress incontinence.*

90 *Exercise promotes sweating, the mechanism by which the body regulates its temperature and eliminates waste products.*

Benefits of exercise for the kidneys

Most people report an increase in the quality of their life when they exercise with any regularity, whether they are in good health or suffering from a major illness. This includes those with kidney and bladder disorders.

HOW EXERCISE CAN HELP

When you exercise regularly, you increase the strength of the heart, lungs and muscles. You are less likely to be overweight and under-fit.

An exercise session improves your mood and feelings of well-being. You become less stressed, feel refreshed and boost your energy levels. Your sense of being in control is greater – especially important if you are living with a medical condition.

Managing high blood pressure and diabetes

Two of the most common causes of kidney disease are high blood pressure and diabetes. Diabetes can damage the nephrons (which filter the blood) in the kidneys because of sugar staying in the blood. High blood pressure can also damage the small blood vessels and lessen the kidneys' filtering capacity. Exercise and a good diet help to reduce and control both of these diseases.

Controlling cholesterol levels

Many people with a high level of cholesterol often combine a fatty diet with very little exercise. Cholesterol levels in the blood are thought to affect kidney function. Scientists report that patients with kidney disease who maintain a reasonable cholesterol level can preserve their renal function for longer than those who do not. Research at the Harvard School of Public Health discovered that women who took care to build concentrated exercise into their schedules two or three times each week cut their risk of gallstones. It is thought that this exercise reduces cholesterol levels in the bile stored in the gall bladder, which produces gallstones. Most gallstones are largely made up of cholesterol.

> *Research suggests that adults with chronic health problems such as high blood pressure or heart disease can reduce their risk of an early death with just 30 minutes of exercise a week.*

Keeping up the water cycle

When we exercise we sweat (see pages 90–91), and this encourages thirst and the replacement of lost fluids through drinking. Drinking lots of water keeps the body properly hydrated and helps keep the various body systems healthy and working properly, not least the kidneys, bladder and urinary tract.

Exercise and weight control

Exercise burns up calories and builds muscles which in turn burn more calories at future exercise sessions.

Aerobic exercise will use stored fat to keep up energy levels and thus help with weight control.

When you exercise, you become more aware of your body and more motivated to make wiser choices over what you eat and drink.

Maintaining muscle tone

Regular activity improves muscle function for everyone, even those who are incapacitated by illness. It is important to exercise regularly to build muscle tone and strength, and increase endurance.

As far as the urinary tract is concerned, exercising the pelvic floor muscles keeps the area toned and in good shape and helps to maintain bladder control.

Protect against injury and trauma

Care should be taken when exercising, as all physical activity carries risks. Contact sports such as rugby or the martial arts can lead to bad injuries, and blows to the kidney area could lead to kidney disease. (See page 53 for details on kidney protection while playing potentially dangerous sports.)

Problems with incontinence

Many exercises and sports increase the pressure on the pelvic floor and sphincter muscles, particularly when bouncing around. Sports associated with high abdominal pressure include basketball and high-impact aerobics. For these reasons they are best avoided if you have a bladder disorder. However, for many people coping with bladder complaints regular exercise is a vital part of their coping strategy – improving morale and self-image as well as increasing and maintaining fitness.

- Stick to low-impact exercises that don't involve any jumping.
- Pee before exercising
- Avoid caffeine for several hours before working out.

It is important not to give up exercise, as one risk factor for incontinence is being overweight.

HEALING MOVEMENT

Tai chi is an ideal exercise for people with kidney or bladder problems. It is low impact, and the gentle rotational movements and breathing techniques have been shown to reduce high blood pressure and lower stress. The waist-turning movements increase the flow of blood and urine through the kidneys, strengthening their function. Even the gentle controlled walking in tai chi has been shown to improve circulation and stimulate the kidney system. Many people with interstitial cystitis – who cannot normally exercise due to the discomfort caused – find that tai chi is gentle enough to perform, and many report a reduction in their most severe symptoms.

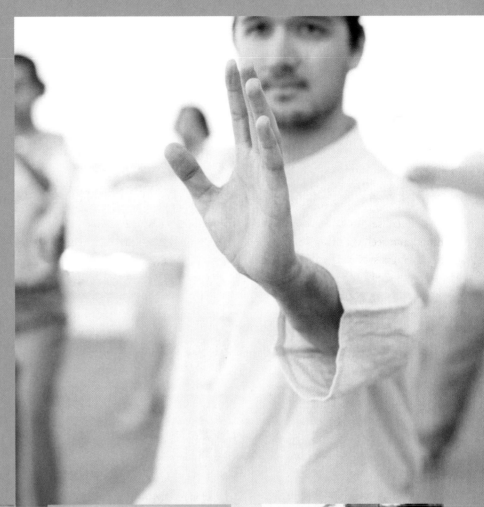

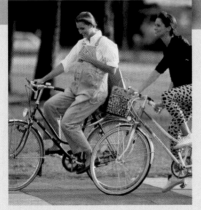

Gently does it!
Cycling during pregnancy can improve the immune system and help to prevent bladder infections. It is good low-impact exercise as long as you stick to flat roads and short rides. You can help keep your back straight by raising the handlebars.

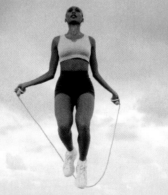

Lifelong fitness
Establishing good health while you are young can prevent complications later in life. A regular exercise routine can help to prevent incontinence and kidney disease caused by high blood pressure, and reduce the risk of cancer.

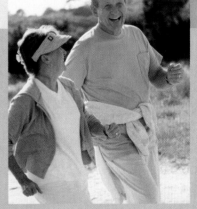

The path to good health
Even a brisk walk is good for you. Just 30 minutes each day will help to reduce body fat, manage weight, lower blood pressure and reduce your risk of developing diabetes. Wear comfortable shoes and always warm up first.

HOW PREGNANCY AFFECTS THE PELVIC FLOOR

Pregnancy and childbirth affect the pelvic floor. The unborn child in the womb exerts constant pressure downwards on to the muscles of the pelvic floor. The uterus grows from being the shape and size of a pear up to 15 times that size, and may be capable of holding as much as 6 litres of fluid.

One of the major hormonal changes that takes place during pregnancy is the increased production of the hormone relaxin, which, as its name suggests, helps to relax all fibres in the body in preparation for childbirth when the baby has to pass through the pelvis and vagina. By the time of birth the pelvic floor is well and truly softened; it is then stretched beyond recognition as the baby is born.

After months of continuous pressure during pregnancy, then over-stretching at

childbirth, it is little wonder that the pelvic floor muscles are not what they were once the child is born. Weak and over-stretched muscles can lose their flexibility for sudden contraction, and a problem with stress incontinence can develop. In really severe cases, lack of muscle tone can lead to a prolapse, when the urethra, bladder or rectal wall protrude into the vaginal area.

What you can do about it

Exercising the pelvic floor muscles before and after giving birth can help to keep muscles toned and supple so that they have more pliability and strength. Thus they will have greater resistance to being over-stretched during childbirth and are more likely to get back into shape after the birth.

WHEN NOT TO EXERCISE

Despite all the good that exercise can do for people with all kinds of medical disorders and

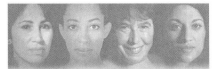

INCONTINENCE AND EXERCISE

Stress incontinence occurs when either the pelvic floor muscles or the sphincter muscle around the urethra are not able to stop urine flow, and so there is involuntary leakage of urine. There are a variety of treatments available to sufferers, depending on the frequency and the severity of the condition. Prescription drugs can help. Vaginal pessaries, diaphragms and even tampons can be used to alter the angle of the urethra. In addition, various mechanical devices can be employed, ranging from pelvic cones (see page 112) to electrical stimulation.

conditions, there are times when regular exercise sessions are not a good idea. These include:

- When you have a heavy cold or flu, because you could put strain on your immune system.
- When you have broken a bone, or torn muscles or ligaments – give your body time to rest and heal.
- Following childbirth get advice on exercises which can be started early without damaging the abdomen.

Take a break

If you are used to regular exercise, it can be difficult – and frustrating – to take time out, but when you are not well exercise is counter-productive and can be harmful. Accept that if you are ill or are feeling run down, your usual exercise routine has to be put on hold. As soon as you are well again, you can resume your normal routine.

Exercise for people with kidney problems

A regular exercise programme has many benefits for people with failing kidneys. Dialysis patients find that exercise can help them to fight symptoms of anaemia and post-transplant patients can speed their rate of recovery.

Although high-impact exercise is usually best avoided by patients undergoing dialysis, some clinics have stationary cycles so that patients can do some gentle exercise while undergoing treatment. Slightly more vigorous exercise can usually be taken the day following treatment. A patient who also has heart problems may be referred to a cardiac rehabilitation specialist.

People who have lost some kidney function typically report feelings of fatigue and low exercise tolerance, which can increase in the first few days of starting to exercise, but this usually dissipates. Exercise can still increase stamina and reduce feelings of anxiety and depression. It can also help to stimulate the immune system.

After a kidney transplant patients are encouraged to begin a regular exercise plan, as it is unhealthy for the new kidney and their general well-being to put on weight. After surgery, modest exercise can help increase strength, regain muscle tone and rebuild the muscles which were cut. It can also reduce the need for medication to lower blood pressure.

- The exercise session does not need to be exhaustive; patients should always start with a few minutes of mobility work and build up their programme gradually and gently.
- To increase heart rate they can walk faster, cycle or just move rhythmically in a small space until they feel their breathing increase.
- Weight training could start off with simply lifting cans of baked beans in each hand, then progress to heavier weights or dumbbells.
- A 12-week programme of gentle activity including walking, cycling and weight training can improve muscle function and walking capacity in patients of any age. A 24-week programme can improve muscle function by 25 per cent.

SIMPLE STEPS TO FITNESS

There are many easy ways to start improving your level of fitness without having to follow a strict exercise regime.

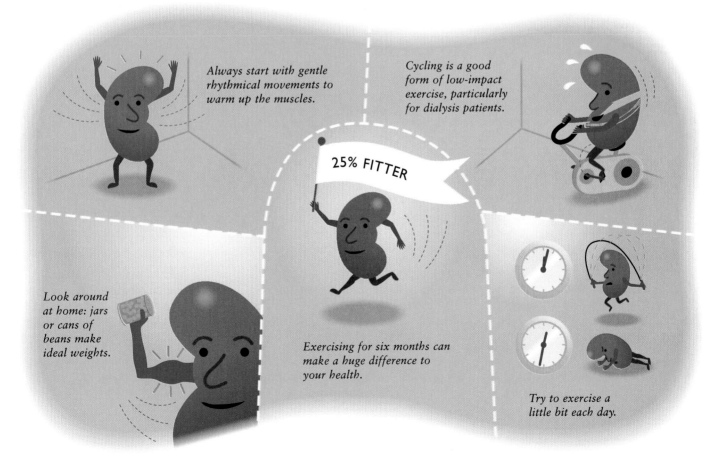

Always start with gentle rhythmical movements to warm up the muscles.

Cycling is a good form of low-impact exercise, particularly for dialysis patients.

25% FITTER

Look around at home: jars or cans of beans make ideal weights.

Exercising for six months can make a huge difference to your health.

Try to exercise a little bit each day.

Pelvic floor exercises

Pelvic floor exercises are designed to strengthen and build up the muscles in the pelvic floor – the muscles that you squeeze to stop the passing of urine or a bowel movement. A strong pelvic floor can help to avoid stress incontinence.

No one can detect when you exercise your pelvic floor muscles, since you are not pulling in on the stomach or your buttocks. The exercises can be done discreetly, anywhere and at any time. This means they can be practised several times a day and yet not interfere with your daily routine.

WHERE ARE THESE MUSCLES?

Your pelvic floor is a sling of muscle which forms the base of the pelvis. In women the pelvic muscles are in two halves – in a figure of eight – that span out on either side of the vaginal, urinary and anal openings; the muscles attach to the pubic bones at the front and to the coccyx (bottom part of the spine) at the back. There are two layers of muscle:

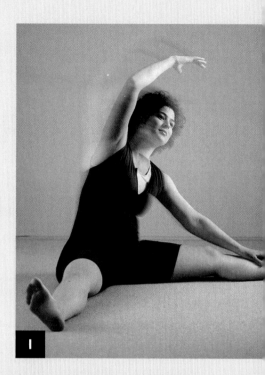

one superficial and the other deep. In men the pelvic muscles run around the anus and the base of the penis.

The link with incontinence

The pelvic floor muscles are usually firm and tense to stop urine leaking out of the bladder. To allow urine to pass, the muscles relax; once the bladder is empty, they tense again.

When the pelvic floor muscles are weak there is less control over this process and urine may leak when you laugh, sneeze, cough or if any pressure is put on the pelvic floor – as when exercising, for example.

Pelvic floor muscles respond to being worked. As they are contracted and released, they become stronger and more pliable. In women, these muscles undergo great stress during a vaginal birth, but all women should aim to keep this area toned. Not only does this reduce the risk of incontinence, it helps during childbirth, and may improve your sex life.

Start by sitting in any comfortable position. When you first try to get in touch with these muscles, kneeling or getting down on all fours may make it easier to locate them. The exercises can be done in any position, as long as you are relaxed.

First, squeeze the muscles around the back passage (all around the anus), then release. Then try to squeeze the muscles around the vagina (the muscles used during sex) and release. Finally, squeeze the muscles you use when you go to the toilet, and release.

Repeat 'back, middle, front', until you have control of these muscles. Gradually increase the frequency with which you perform them.

---

positive health tips

Tips to bear in mind

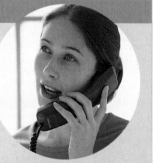

- Pregnant women, new mothers and women trying to conceive should try to perform at least 50 'holds' a day. Ideally, this should be from the first day of pregnancy onwards.

- The hardest thing about pelvic floor exercises is remembering to do them. Make a connection between something you do regularly and a reminder to do your exercises. For instance, if you pick up the phone several times a day, you could use that as your cue to discreetly perform a few pelvic floor squeezes.

- One of the best ways to remember to do the exercises is to perform them every time you go to the toilet. Wait until you have emptied your bladder – don't, as is sometimes suggested, perform the exercise in mid-flow.

- Get your partner to test the strength of your squeeze next time you are making love. He can let you know when muscle tone improves.

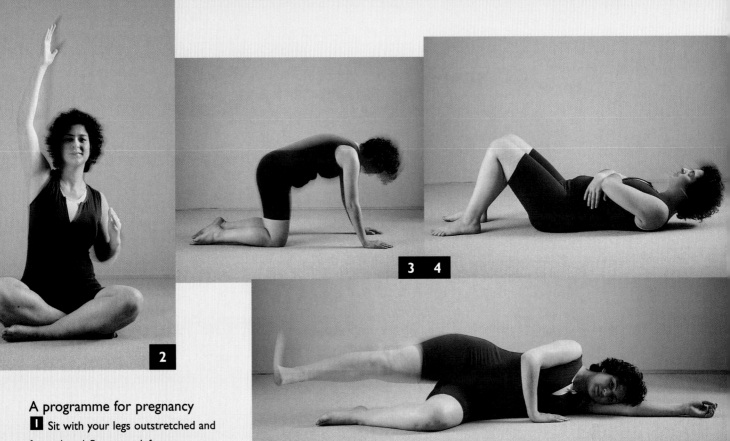

2

A programme for pregnancy

1 Sit with your legs outstretched and feet relaxed. Rest your left arm on your left leg, breathe out and circle your head with your right arm. Repeat five times, then repeat using your left arm. This loosens the pelvic floor area.

2 Sit with your legs crossed and back straight. Stretch up first one arm then the other towards the ceiling, feeling the stretch in your sides. Stretch each arm in turn five times.

3 Kneel on all fours with your back parallel to the floor. Inhale, and as you

3 **4**

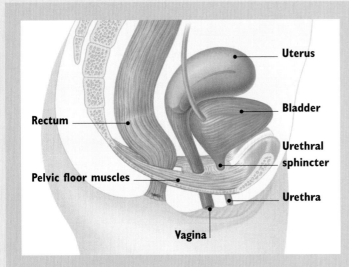

5

exhale curve your back up towards the ceiling. Slowly straighten so that is it is parallel to the floor again. Repeat five times. This strengthens the abdominal muscles and improves overall posture.

4 Lie on your back with your knees bent and feet flat on the floor. Cross your arms on your stomach, breathe out and raise your head for a count of

three. Lower your head back to the floor. Repeat five times. This strengthens the abdominal muscles, preventing weakness in this area after the birth.

5 Lie on your left side with your left arm outstretched. Breathe out as you raise your right leg so that it is parallel to the floor. Repeat five times, then change legs. This strengthens the hip and buttocks.

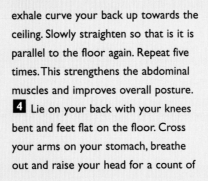

Uterus

Bladder

Rectum

Urethral sphincter

Pelvic floor muscles

Urethra

Vagina

IDENTIFYING THE PELVIC FLOOR MUSCLES

To perform pelvic floor exercises correctly, you must first be sure you are exercising the right muscles. Identify these by starting to urinate, then deliberately stopping; as you stop, focus on which muscles are being used. Another way is to insert a finger in the vagina and then squeeze as hard as possible; there is a feeling of pressure around the finger when the pelvic floor muscles are in use.

Why we sweat when exercising

Sweating has two major functions. When the temperature rises – due to exercise or hot weather – sweating cools the body down. Sweating is also one of the principal ways of expelling water and waste products from the body.

Sweating, together with panting, is the body's way of maintaining an appropriate temperature. When the temperature rises, our sweating mechanism comes into play to return the body to its normal temperature of around 37°C. The body's temperature is affected not only by external heat in the atmosphere but also by internal heat created by exercising and eating.

We sweat continuously, even though we may only become aware of this when the sweating significantly increases – due to vigorous exercise, for instance.

Sweating is also a way of expelling water and other waste products from the body. Water is also lost as urine from the kidneys and bladder, as water vapour and carbon dioxide from the lungs, and as waste matter from the intestines.

Where we sweat

The average person has approximately 2.6 million sweat glands in their skin. A sweat gland is essentially a long coiled duct in the dermis layer of the skin. The coiled part is where the sweat is produced, and the end of the duct is the opening, or pore, on the skin's surface. There are two types of sweat glands: the eccrine glands and the apocrine glands.

- Eccrine glands are found all over the body, except the lips, nipples and external genital organs. They are in particularly high numbers on the palms of the hands, the soles of the feet and the forehead.
- Apocrine glands are mostly confined to the armpits and anal-genital area. They don't become active until puberty, unlike eccrine glands, which are active from birth. Apocrine glands end in hair follicles rather than pores.

What is sweat made of?

Sweat from the eccrine glands is primarily water with some sodium and chloride and a low level of potassium. It is these chemicals that make sweaty skin taste salty. Sweat from the apocrine glands also contains proteins and fatty acids, which make it thicker. When these proteins and acids react with the bacteria on hair and skin, a distinctive odour is produced.

HOW SWEATING HELPS US TO COOL DOWN

When we perspire, the water that rises to the skin's surface evaporates, removing excess heat and cooling us down. Heat is also lost directly from the skin and via the respiratory surfaces of the lungs.

Air heavily laden with moisture will not enable the body to cool as efficiently as air that is dryer.

Game, sweat and match
A tennis player swops his sweat-sodden shirt for a fresh, dry one to allow the sweat on his skin to evaporate and so cool him down. His first shirt was so wet that it was blocking the evaporation of water from the surface of the skin and causing him to overheat.

The level of humidity in the air has a direct effect on how quickly water on the skin is able to evaporate, and so how effectively sweating is able to cool you down.

Wiping off sweat during exercise interferes with this natural evaporation and cooling process, as does spraying lots of water onto the skin in an effort to cool down.

Sweating in normal circumstances – in a hot environment or during hard exercise – will not normally cause serious dehydration problems. Overheating, however, can cause symptoms such as light-headedness, nausea and muscle cramping.

Moving to a desert or tropical country can increase sweat loss to up to 3 litres an hour in as little as six weeks.

REPLACING WATER LOSS BROUGHT ON BY SWEATING

Because sweating means you are losing water and chemicals, it is important to replace lost fluids. If you don't, you will suffer the symptoms of dehydration (see pages 69–71), and urine will become more concentrated: this can result in kidney stones.

Relying on thirst is an inaccurate measure of whether you are dehydrated, particularly in children and older people, who often don't feel thirsty. Sip regularly throughout the day. You should drink 8–10 glasses per day, and more when you exercise. Heavy exercise, especially in hot or humid conditions, causes a sweat loss of around a litre an hour.

Sports drink manufacturers claim that their combinations of fluid and special additives will rehydrate you more quickly than plain water, and improve sporting performance as well. In fact, this is generally only necessary for athletes doing extended exercise as extreme as 50–80km runs or 160km cycle rides. Water is plentiful, cheap and good for you, so drink that instead.

Experts disagree on whether the sodium, chloride and potassium lost in sweat needs to be replaced. Most say that is rare for the loss of these chemicals to create an imbalance in the blood so great that it needs to be rectified. Some, however, assert that intense exercise and sweating can cause a calcium depletion that needs to be rectified by taking extra calcium through food or supplements.

COLD SWEATS

It is not only heat and strenuous exercise that can make you perspire. Sweating can also be brought on by nervousness or anxiety, or a combination of both. This 'cold sweat' is part of the classic 'fight or flight' response to an extreme situation. One of the effects of this 'all systems go' response is that the body produces heat that needs to be disposed of. It is because sweating brought on by nervousness is not always accompanied by a rise in temperature that this sweating is referred to as a cold sweat.

CHOOSING EXERCISE GEAR

When exercising, wear clothing that allows sweat to do its job of keeping your body from overheating by evaporating off the surface of the skin and dispersing in the air. This is equally important for underwear as

Are creatine supplements a good idea?

Creatine is an amino acid (protein) produced naturally by the liver. It is also found in meat and fish, and is sold in powder or pill form as a supplement in health stores. They have become popular with athletes as a way of bulking up muscles, by allowing users to recover more quickly after exercise. While there is no evidence that creatine has adverse long-term side effects, nor is there much proof that it does not. It may impair the ability to sweat properly and may damage the kidneys or liver in the long term. Many doctors conclude that until more is known about the effect of creatine supplements they should be approached with caution, and avoided by pregnant and breastfeeding women, children and teenagers.

ASK THE EXPERT

for outer clothes. Fabrics should be lightweight and porous – that is, have tiny gaps in the weave to allow air into and moisture out of the material. Fabric made from natural fibres such as cotton fall into this category, as do many synthetic fabrics specially designed for sports and exercise, to have 'breathable' or 'evaporative' qualities.

If you are exercising in the sun, bright colours, especially white, will keep you cooler, because they reflect light from the sun; dark colours soak up the heat, as do soft colours – even pale ones – so they are best avoided.

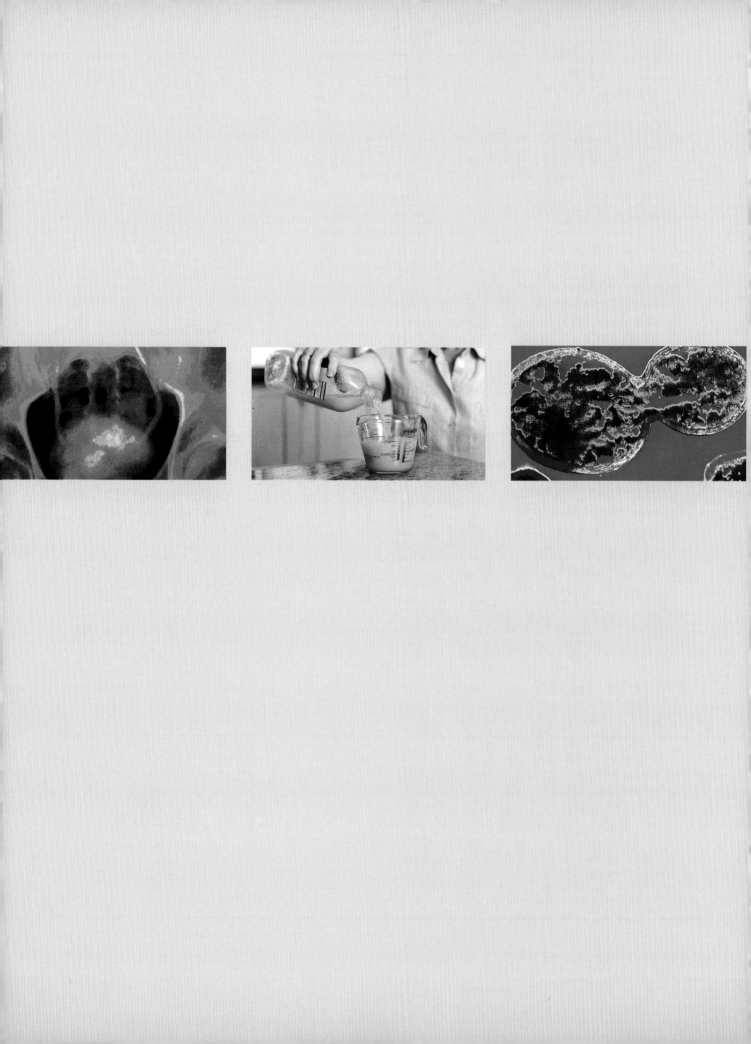

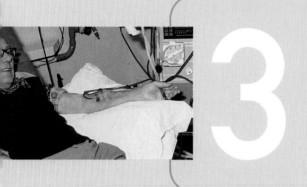

3

What happens when things go wrong

Knowing what can go wrong

Our kidneys and urinary system fulfil an essential role in cleansing the blood and excreting waste products from the body. It's important to know how the normal functioning of this organ system can go wrong so you can help the doctor make the correct diagnosis.

COMMON PROBLEMS

Conditions that challenge the normal functioning of the kidney and urinary tract are very common and symptoms can have a major impact on your health. In the UK, 60 people per million die each year of diseases of the kidneys and urinary tract, and an estimated 1 in 12 of all doctor consultations are related to such difficulties. Furthermore, many people's daily lives are disrupted by conditions such as incontinence, which, although not life-threatening, can severely affect day-to-day living.

CONGENITAL CONDITIONS

The development of the kidneys and urinary tract in the embryo involves the coordinated growth of structures from different origins, and therefore it is not surprising that things go wrong occasionally. Many conditions are minor – with little or no significant effect on the function of the kidneys – and so are rarely detected. For example, some congenital

MORE COMMON

ENLARGED PROSTATE GLAND
10,000 PER 100,000 MEN AT AGE 70 (1 IN 10)
Approximately 10 per cent of men aged 70 and upwards have symptoms of incontinence arising from an enlarged prostate gland requiring medical advice and treatment.

INCONTINENCE
Each year, 5–6 per cent of UK adults experience urinary incontinence – that's between 1 in 17 and 1 in 20. Only an estimate is possible because so many cases go unreported.

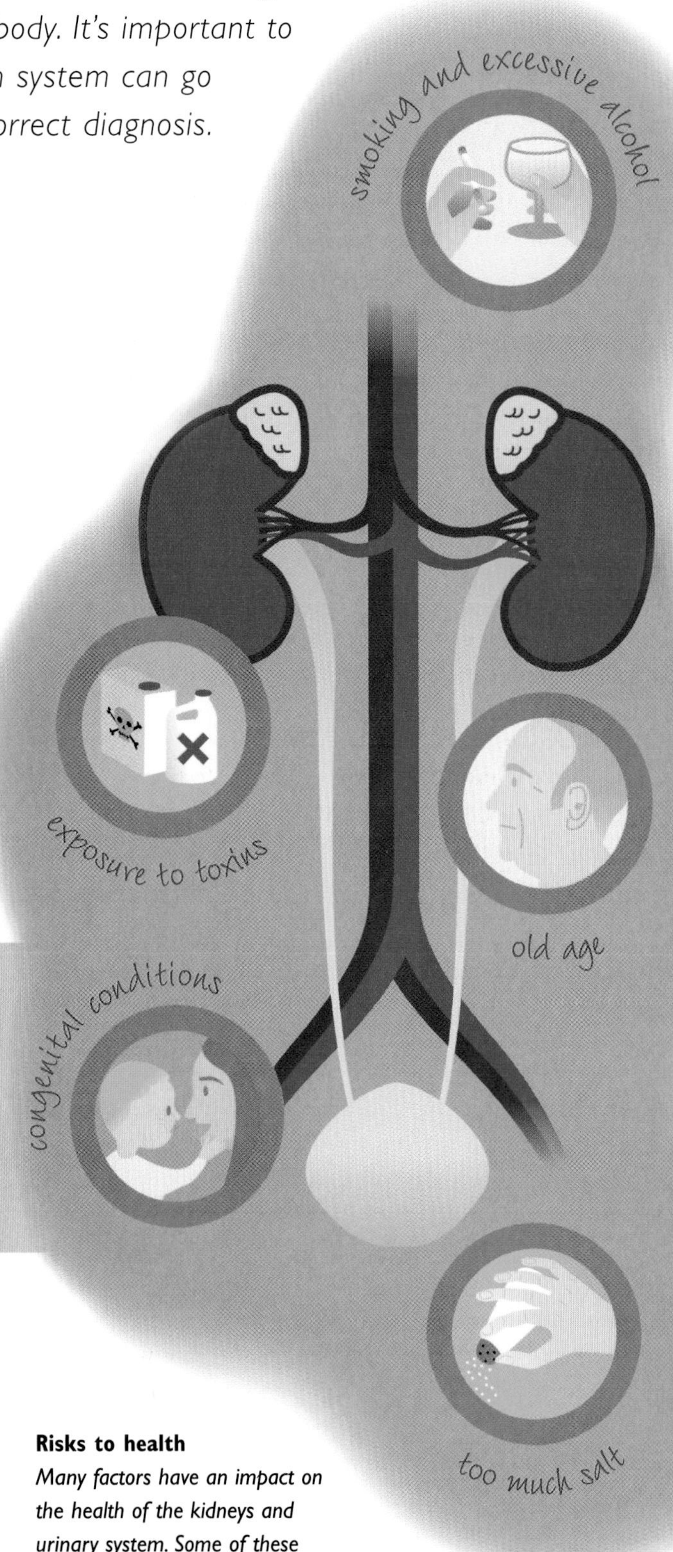

defects (such as duplication of the ureters) can cause urine to back up from the bladder to the kidneys, which predisposes an individual to recurrent urinary tract infections. Major congenital abnormalities – those that do alter the ability of the kidneys to clear body wastes and balance fluids – are usually apparent at birth or in early childhood. They are also increasingly being detected before birth, with the improved quality and accuracy of ultrasound scanning in pregnancy, and this often results in earlier treatment of those affected.

smoking and excessive alcohol

exposure to toxins

old age

congenital conditions

too much salt

Risks to health
Many factors have an impact on the health of the kidneys and urinary system. Some of these are illustrated here, together with figures indicating how common these problems are in the UK.

INFECTION

Infections are very common and, in the vast majority of cases, mild and easily treated. Most infections result from bacteria ascending into the bladder from the outside, and are more common in women than in men because women have a much shorter urethra, making the distance the bacteria have to travel much smaller. Advancing age also increases the risk of urinary tract infection.

STONES

Kidney stones can cause dramatic and sudden pain, usually in the back and flanks. A common symptom is blood in the urine (haematuria). Men are four times more likely to develop stones than women, but the reasons for this are not at all clear. Anyone who has had stones diagnosed in the past is likely to have them again, so preventative measures become important. These include keeping adequately hydrated in hot climates, treating infections promptly, and keeping a check on calcium levels in the urine.

TUMOURS

Although very much less common than infections and stones, tumours of the kidney and urinary tract account for a significant proportion of all types of cancer. Men are

Honeymoon cystitis is a myth, isn't it?

The onset of sexual activity does increase a woman's chances of developing cystitis. Women are more prone to developing bladder infections in general than men, because a woman's urethra is shorter than a man's, meaning that bacteria from outside the body can enter the bladder more easily. During sex a woman's urethra is pulled and stretched, so bacteria can be 'pushed up' into the bladder, resulting in symptoms of frequency, urgency and a burning pain on passing urine. The risks of this occurring are reduced if simple measures are followed such as emptying the bladder after sex and always wiping from front to back.

ASK THE EXPERT

is not cleared. Such an obstruction can be caused either by stones and tumours or as a result of pressure from structures close by which become enlarged for some reason. For example, in men, enlargement of the prostate gland often obstructs the flow of urine, while in women, an enlarged uterus can cause urinary obstruction or may reduce the capacity of the bladder by pressing on it.

LESS COMMON

URINARY TRACT INFECTIONS 5000 PER 100,000 (1 IN 20) Mostly women. Again, this figure is very approximate, since there is no accurate centralised database for the number of cases of urinary tract infections (including cystitis) in the UK.	KIDNEY STONES 100 PER 10,000 (1 IN 100) Most patients with stones are aged 20–50; stones occur more often in men than in women.	CANCER AT 70 YEARS OLD: PROSTATE: 350 PER 100,000 MEN (1 IN 285) BLADDER: 150 PER 100,000 (1 IN 666) KIDNEY: 50 PER 100,000 (1 IN 2000) The numbers increase with age.	WAITING FOR A KIDNEY TRANSPLANT 10 PER 100,000 (1 IN 10,000) About 1350 kidney transplants take place in the UK each year. There are about 6000 UK citizens waiting for a kidney transplant.

at particular risk, as all types of tumour that arise in the urinary tract are more common in men than in women. The prostate gland – in men only, at the bladder's base – is the most common source of urinary tract cancers.

OBSTRUCTION

The urinary tract acts as a waste pipe for disposing of water-soluble toxins from the body and – like any pipe – it can get blocked. This leads to back-pressure on the kidneys that can cause permanent damage if the blockage

TRAUMA

The urinary tract, like other soft structures in the body, can be damaged in an accident such as a car crash. A full bladder may rupture if exposed to great force. If the pelvis is fractured, the ureters (that carry urine from kidneys to bladder) or the urethra (the outflow pipe from the bladder) may be torn. The urinary tract may also receive traumatic damage as a complication of surgery. Damage to the ureters and bladder is a well-recognised, though rare, complication of abdominal surgery.

RISK FACTORS

Most disorders of the kidneys and urinary tract have associated risk factors which increase the chances of developing that condition. A GP will try to establish any predisposing risk factors in a patient, as part of taking a medical history. Some predisposing risk factors, such as age, are unavoidable. However, many risk factors can be modified by carefully thought out changes in lifestyle.

GENETIC AND HEREDITARY FACTORS

Children can inherit sets or combinations of genes from their parents that predispose them to certain illnesses. Polycystic kidney disease, for example, is the result of a single faulty gene being passed from one generation to the next. As more is discovered about the functions of the millions of genes that make up the human genome, it will become possible to predict from birth the disorders to which any one person is particularly susceptible. This information will enable each person to take whatever appropriate action they can to reduce the likelihood of them developing these disorders.

AGE

Ageing is a risk factor for many disorders of the kidneys and urinary tract. There are several reasons for this.

- There is an accumulation of damage from wear and tear on organs and on individual cells. Most organs have far more capacity to carry out their function than is normally required. This means they can continue to do their job even if disease reduces their efficiency. As organs age, this spare capacity diminishes and so organs are less able to adjust to a condition that causes damage to, for example, the kidneys.

- Over a lifetime the cells that make up the organs of the urinary tract divide many times. This process can sometimes lead to the creation of faulty 'mutated' cells. An accumulation of faulty cells causes a decline in the ability of the cells to perform their function. Damage to the genetic code may also lead to uncontrolled cell growth and division, which results in cancer.

- The strength of the support tissues that hold organs in place declines with age. This is particularly significant in women. The female reproductive organs and bladder are supported by a group of muscles and ligaments that make up the 'pelvic floor'. Advancing age, childbirth and lower levels of oestrogen after the menopause can lead to a weakness of these support structures, which may contribute to incontinence and prolapse.

LIFESTYLE

Smoking, and drinking too much alcohol, are risk factors for many kidney and bladder diseases, especially cancer.

A healthy balanced diet and regular, moderate exercise allows the body to maintain resistance to infection. Being overweight increases susceptibility to high blood pressure and diabetes – both of which damage the kidneys – and also to incontinence.

Sexual behaviour can also have an effect. Sexually transmitted infections can not only give rise to pain on passing urine but can also scar the urinary tract, affecting its function long after other symptoms have passed. This risk is greatly reduced by the use of barrier contraception.

OCCUPATION

There are a number of environmental chemical toxins to which workers in particular occupations are exposed, that can result in damage to the kidneys and urinary tract. In the past, for example, workers in the dye and rubber industries risked developing bladder cancer. Fortunately, in many countries there are now health and safety measures in place to reduce occupation-related risks.

Eat fresh food for healthy kidneys
Fresh food not only contains higher levels of essential vitamins and minerals, but also avoids the high salt content of packaged and fast foods. Over time, high levels of salt intake can damage the kidneys and lead to high blood pressure.

Who's who – urological and renal health experts

Urinary disorders are common, and can often be treated by your own GP. Even if a specialist is needed, a GP can combine knowledge of the case and of local medical services to refer each patient to the most appropriate specialist.

GENERAL PRACTITIONER

Many diseases of the kidneys and urinary tract can be diagnosed and treated by a GP. A well-taken history, physical examination and simple initial investigations can often direct a GP to a problem's cause.

CONTINENCE ADVISER

A GP normally refers patients with urinary continence problems to a continence adviser. At the continence adviser's clinic a patient will be assessed, and then advised on all aspects of his or her condition and treatment. This may include instruction in pelvic floor exercises, bladder retraining, self-catheterisation and other necessary skills.

GYNAECOLOGIST

This is a specialist concerned with the study, diagnosis and treatment of diseases of the female reproductive tract. Because the reproductive organs and lower urinary tract are so close together in women, changes in the support of the pelvic organs often affect both systems. When appropriate, therefore, women who have symptoms such as incontinence may see a gynaecologist. Gynaecologists with an interest in urology are termed urogynaecologists.

NEPHROLOGIST

The nephrologist investigates and treats diseases affecting the kidney. He or she is a physician, not a surgeon, but works closely with urologists and renal transplant surgeons. For example, a urologist may surgically remove kidney stones from a patient, but a nephrologist will find out why the stones formed and may give medication to prevent further stone formation. Nephrologists run dialysis programmes for patients with renal failure.

RENAL TRANSPLANT SURGEON

The renal transplant surgeon performs kidney transplants and is responsible for retrieving kidneys from organ donors. They may also perform operations to enable patients with kidney failure to receive dialysis. Renal

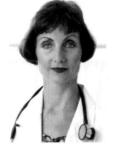

UROLOGIST

This is a hospital-based specialist concerned with the study, diagnosis and treatment of diseases of the kidneys, urinary tract and the male reproductive system. A urologist is a surgeon, trained to perform operations but also to treat patients by administering drugs, working closely with a nephrologist. Urologists also perform tests to assess bladder function and may treat patients with impotence.

transplant surgeons are usually skilled in another surgical specialty too – urology, vascular surgery or liver transplant surgery – and each kidney transplant unit is staffed by a team of renal transplant surgeons, where each one has a different second surgical speciality.

DIALYSIS TECHNICIAN

The dialysis or renal technician maintains the haemodialysis machines used to treat patients with acute and chronic kidney failure. The majority of their work will be in the dialysis unit of a hospital, but dialysis technicians may also be responsible for establishing some patients on home haemodialysis.

TRANSPLANT COORDINATOR

The transplant coordinator is responsible for coordinating organ retrieval for transplantation. This includes the task of obtaining consent for organ donation from relatives whose loved one has died. Some coordinators are based in transplant units, others in intensive care units. Some have responsibility for organising donation from living donors.

FINDING OUT WHAT IS WRONG

Today's doctors are armed with an impressive array of sophisticated equipment – including X-rays, ultrasound and computed tomography (CT) scanners – for investigating the many causes of urinary symptoms. At the same time, the function of the kidneys and bladder can be assessed accurately in a variety of ways, from simple blood tests to complex urodynamic testing.

In the early stages of investigation it is usual to obtain some images of the kidney on plain abdominal X-ray film (KUB) or by ultrasound. Thereafter more specialised tests may be employed to investigate continuing concerns.

Medical history and examination

The most important clues as to what may be wrong come from a well-taken medical history and physical examination. This forms the basis from which all subsequent tests and investigations can be planned and prioritised in order to pinpoint a diagnosis.

THE PATIENT'S MEDICAL HISTORY – THE FIRST STEP TO DIAGNOSIS

The patient will need to describe to the doctor all of the physical symptoms experienced, as the patient is the only person who can describe them accurately. The importance of a good description should not be underestimated: even in this age of hi-tech modern medicine, this is invaluable in directing a doctor to the causes of any problems.

Current symptoms

The doctor will want to know the nature of the symptoms, the length of time the patient has noticed them, the site, the number of times a day the patient is affected and for how long. The patient should also mention anything that seems to worsen or improve the symptoms, and how the symptoms impact on normal daily activities. Failure to mention important information could slow down or misdirect the diagnostic process.

THE PHYSICAL EXAMINATION

This will have started from the moment the doctor first greets the patient. A great deal of useful information can be gained from simple observation.
• Are there signs of obvious pain?
• Does the patient look pale and anaemic?
• Are there signs of weight loss?
A general physical examination will include an assessment of pulse, blood pressure and temperature. It may also include the head and chest if there are particular signs that the doctor is alerted to look for as a result of the patient's medical history.

Abdominal examination

The purpose of this is to detect any masses that may be present and to get an idea of their size and where they may originate. The presence of any tenderness and its

Know your symptoms

Pain It is important to describe the nature, site, duration and severity of pain, as well as activities that make it better or worse.

Swelling Swelling may occur in kidney diseases that lead to water and salt retention. Site, duration and severity are important factors.

Haematuria The presence of blood in the urine is always a significant symptom. It may be visible to the naked eye (frank haematuria) or present in such small amounts that it is only detectable by urinalysis (microscopic haematuria).

Itching Itching all over the body may be a significant symptom, especially if combined with other signs and symptoms. It can occur in kidney diseases where toxins are not properly cleared from the body.

Hesitancy This is a difficulty and delay in starting to pass urine. It usually occurs in the presence of urinary obstruction.

Poor flow rate This is a reduction in the normal stream of urine, caused by a partial blockage or weak bladder contractions. It is more often found in men, as the result of enlargement of the prostate gland, and occasionally in women, usually as the result of scarring from previous bladder surgery.

Incontinence* This is the involuntary loss of urine from the bladder. It should be described in terms of how frequently it occurs, under what circumstances, how often protective pads need to be changed and how it affects social function.

Urinary frequency* This is the frequent passage of small quantities of urine. The total volume passed per day is usually normal however.

Polyuria This is the passage of larger than normal volumes of urine during the course of a day and is usually accompanied by excessive fluid intake (polydipsia). This may be the result of diabetes or a behavioural problem caused by excessive drinking.

Urgency* Urgency is a sudden desire to pass urine which, if ignored, may result in incontinence.

Frequency Frequency is defined as regularly passing urine more than eight times during the course of a day.

Nocturia* Nocturia describes the need to pass urine with increased frequency at night. It is counted as significant if it happens on a regular basis.

* Symptoms of urinary frequency, urgency, nocturia and incontinence are most clearly described by use of a frequency volume chart (see page 100).

Urine analyis

Any physical examination should include an assessment of a fresh urine sample by urinalysis. A multiple test stick – a chemically coated strip – is dipped into the urine sample; the stick will change colour to demonstrate the presence of protein, sugar or blood in the urine.

location is another important finding. The kidneys lie on either side of the spine at the back of the abdomen and are usually examined with one hand pushing upwards from the back, and the other hand on the front of the abdomen. The kidneys cannot usually be felt unless they are enlarged. The lower abdomen is examined for the presence of an enlarged bladder, which may indicate urinary retention.

Rectal and vaginal examinations

For men in particular, a rectal examination is extremely important, as it allows the prostate gland to be felt for enlargement. This is a common finding in men over the age of 50 who complain of poor urinary stream, and can be the result of either benign or malignant growths.

In women, the close proximity of the reproductive organs to the urinary tract means that it is important to rule out a gynaecological cause of urinary symptoms that result in a reduction of bladder capacity and urinary frequency. An example of this would be an enlarged uterus pressing on the bladder.

The female reproductive organs are assessed by means of a vaginal examination, in which the fingers of one hand gently push up on the uterus and other pelvic organs from below, while the other hand pushes down on the abdomen. This allows the size of the uterus to be estimated. Furthermore, the examination can determine whether the pelvic organs are well supported or are 'coming down' the vagina. Known as pelvic organ prolapse, this is related to weakness in the pelvic floor and urinary incontinence.

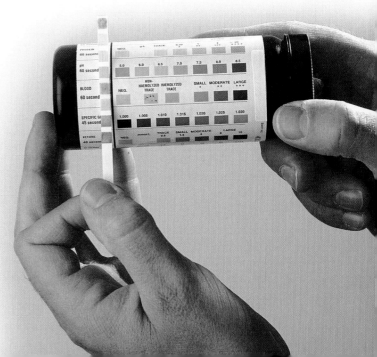

Initial tests

Initial investigation into problems of the kidneys, bladder and urinary tract will normally include a dipstick test for blood and protein in the urine, a midstream urine sample to look for infection, and basic blood tests to check overall kidney function.

BLOOD TEST

A blood test will include measurement of urea and creatinine in the blood, both of which are eliminated from the blood if the kidneys are functioning normally. The higher the level of either substance in the blood, the worse the overall kidney function. In early kidney failure, where blood creatinine does not rise much, a more accurate test of overall kidney disease is used. Known as the 'creatinine clearance test', this measures the amount of blood that is cleaned by the kidney in one day, and is the main test used to monitor kidney function.

Since the functions of the kidney include regulation of acid/alkali balance and levels of potassium, and phosphate and uric acid elimination, measurement of these substances in the blood also contributes to the overall assessment of kidney function. With worsening kidney failure, the blood becomes more acid and levels of phosphate and uric acid rise.

MIDSTREAM URINE SPECIMEN (MSU)

This is a basic investigation for anyone with urinary symptoms. A fresh sample of urine is collected from the middle of the stream in a sterile container, then examined under a microscope for evidence of blood (microscopic haematuria) or bacteria and pus, which suggest urinary tract infection. The sample is then cultured for several days in an agar dish. If bacteria grow, they can be identified and tested against a variety of antibiotics to determine their sensitivity. In this way the most appropriate antibiotic can be chosen to treat the infection.

MEASURING URINARY INCONTINENCE

A simple pad test provides an accurate way of estimating the amount of leakage from the bladder due to incontinence. It is performed by asking the patient to wear a pre-weighed incontinence pad for a set period of time – say one hour – after which the pad is weighed again to determine the amount of urine that has leaked. During this test the patient would typically be asked to drink 500ml (just under a pint) of water and perform a series of activities designed to provoke incontinence.

Filling out a frequency volume chart

A frequency volume chart (as shown right) is a tool for studying bladder function in greater detail. All fluid taken into the body over a three to five-day period is accurately measured, as is all the urine that passes out of it during that time. The chart itself takes the form of a time sheet. The times that various volumes of fluid enter or leave the body are recorded, plus episodes of incontinence (W) and pad usage. The chart does not reveal the causes of incontinence, but it can convey a lot of useful information.

- It gives an idea of the pattern of fluid intake throughout the day. Often, simple advice on reducing fluid intake at certain times of the day, such as just before bedtime, can bring about a great improvement in symptoms.
- The capacity of the bladder can be gauged, and the frequency of passing urine during the daytime and at night can be clearly seen.
- The chart gives an idea of the severity of any incontinence.

	Monday		Tuesday	
	In	Out	In	Out
6am	250			
7am				
8am		50		
9am	250	150		
10am				
11am	175	100		
12				25
1pm				
2pm	180	W		
3pm				
4pm				
5pm	300	200		
6pm				190
7pm		75		
8pm				
9pm	125	100		
10pm				150
11pm				
12				
1am				
2am		W		
3am				
4am				
5am				175
Waking	6am		7.30am	
Retiring	12.30am		11.30pm	
Pad usage	3		1	

Urodynamic testing

This is a collective term for tests which look at how the lower urinary tract (the bladder and urethra) is functioning. A patient would not normally expect to have all these tests performed, but rather a selection of them, depending on the patient's symptoms and medical history.

UROFLOWMETRY

This simple test measures the flow rate of the urinary stream. Before starting, the bladder must be reasonably full. The patient is asked to pass urine into a special commode, which measures both rate of flow and the total volume passed. This test is useful for men who are suspected of having an enlarged prostate gland and who may complain of a poor, prolonged flow as a result.

RESIDUAL URINE MEASUREMENT

If the bladder doesn't completely empty each time urine is passed, a residual pool can collect at the bottom of the bladder. This becomes stagnant and may lead to urinary tract infection. Residual volume is measured by inserting a catheter into the bladder after passing urine and measuring what comes out, or by using an ultrasound scanner to measure the size of the bladder and the volume of urine left inside. Small amounts are not significant but chances of infection are increased if there is regularly more than 100ml of urine left in the bladder after voiding.

SUBTRACTED CYSTOMETRY

This test measures the strength and frequency of contractions generated by the bladder muscle under different situations and stimuli. Pressure-measuring catheters placed inside the patient's bladder and rectum monitor the bladder muscle throughout the test.

- Firstly, the bladder is slowly filled with sterile fluid.
- Then the bladder is 'provoked' by stimuli such as running a tap or washing the hands.
- The patient is asked to cough or to jump up and down.
- `The patient is asked to empty the bladder. If outflow from the bladder is partially blocked or obstructed the bladder muscle will have to generate a lot of pressure to squeeze urine past the blockage. This is most commonly seen in men with an enlarged prostate gland.

MICTURATING CYSTOURETHROGRAPHY

This is an X-ray based test in which the bladder is filled with a contrast solution that shows up its position and shape. Rather than take a single static picture, the person performing the test screens the bladder as the bladder is emptied. As the passage of contrast solution out of the bladder is followed, the purpose of the test is to see if any of the solution squirts back up the wrong way, towards the kidneys. Known as vesicoureteric reflux, this can lead to recurrent infections of the kidney, scarring and long-term damage. This test might also be used to show up any abnormal connections between the bladder and other organs that are close, such as the bowel.

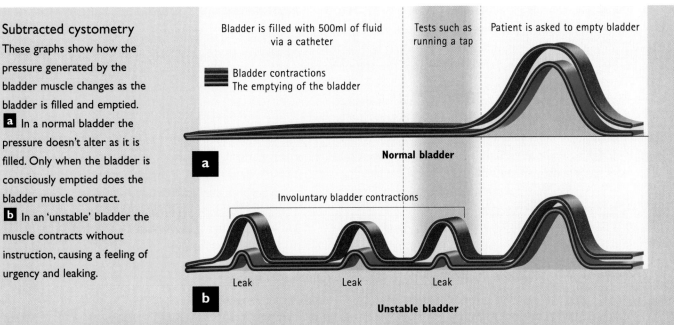

Subtracted cystometry
These graphs show how the pressure generated by the bladder muscle changes as the bladder is filled and emptied.
a In a normal bladder the pressure doesn't alter as it is filled. Only when the bladder is consciously emptied does the bladder muscle contract.
b In an 'unstable' bladder the muscle contracts without instruction, causing a feeling of urgency and leaking.

Bladder is filled with 500ml of fluid via a catheter

Tests such as running a tap

Patient is asked to empty bladder

Bladder contractions
The emptying of the bladder

Normal bladder

Involuntary bladder contractions

Leak   Leak   Leak

Unstable bladder

Imaging tests

The successful diagnosis and treatment of many urological and renal conditions has been greatly advanced over the last few decades through the development of techniques such as ultrasound, MRI and CT scanning.

PLAIN ABDOMINAL X-RAY OF KIDNEY-URETER-BLADDER AREA (KUB)

A simple X-ray of the full length of the abdomen that includes the kidneys, ureters and bladder is known as a KUB. The technique involves irradiation and is used sparingly in patients of an age when they might want to have children. This simple technique is a good method of detecting stones in any part of the urinary tract.

INTRAVENOUS PYELOGRAM/UROGRAM (IVP, IVU)

More sophisticated than the simple X-ray, this method uses an X-ray contrast material injected into a vein. The material is removed from the blood by the kidney and highlights the kidneys, ureters and bladder.

What is it used for?

The technique is undertaken to show the precise anatomical detail of the kidney, the urinary collecting system and the drainage from the kidney into the bladder. It is of particular value in the diagnosis of stone disease, reflux (back-flow) nephropathy, tumours and obstruction. It can also show up whether or not the bladder is being emptied completely, and how much urine is remaining.

How does it work?

The patient receives an intravenous injection of 50–100ml of a clear, fluid, X-ray contrast material that is opaque to X-rays. It is rapidly removed from the bloodstream by the kidneys. X-ray pictures are taken at specific times: for example, just before the injection and immediately afterwards, then at 5, 10, 15 and 25 minutes afterwards, then at 45 minutes – just before and after the bladder is emptied. By doing this, the passage of the X-ray contrast material is caught at various stages during its removal from the bloodstream and collection in the bladder.

Are there any adverse effects?

It is normal to feel a little warm and flushed after the injection, but otherwise there is no significant discomfort. There is a risk of kidney damage – usually reversible – if

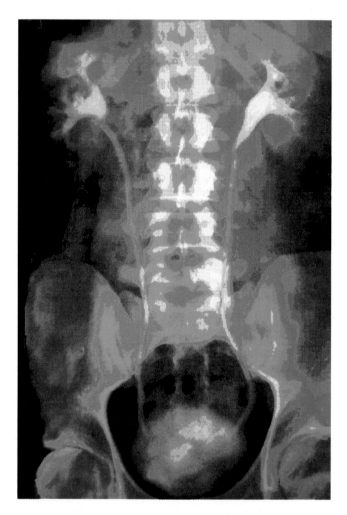

A coloured intravenous urogram of the abdomen
From the kidneys (shown in yellow, top left and right), the ureters extend to the bladder (green and red, bottom centre). The lower spine and pelvic girdle are both shown in blue.

high doses of the X-ray contrast material are given, and this is particularly true in patients with diabetes mellitus, multiple myeloma and significant pre-existing kidney impairment. Kidney damage from the X-ray contrast can be minimised by ensuring a high fluid intake before and immediately after the examination. There is a very small risk of an allergic reaction to the X-ray contrast material; this can be serious but is extremely rare.

ULTRASOUND

Ultrasound uses high-frequency sound waves to obtain an image of internal organs. The procedure is quick, economical, safe and painless.

Ultrasound can be used to measure kidney size accurately. This is important because small kidneys are associated with long-standing chronic kidney disease. Ultrasound can also check for obstruction as a possible cause of impaired kidney function, and is of great value in the investigation of cysts. A type of sonography known as Doppler ultrasound can be used to assess blood flow to the kidneys – of particular value in patients with suspected narrowing of the main renal artery.

A probe is placed on the surface of the skin and a beam of high-frequency ultrasound waves passes into the body and is reflected from the organs within. The reflected waves can be formatted to produce a picture of the internal organs. The anatomical detail provided by ultrasound is not as precise as some of the other techniques that involve irradiation (see below).

RADIONUCLIDE SCANNING

It is possible to make a variety of complex substances radioactive by tagging them to a tiny amount of a radioactive substance such as technetium. If the agent that has been radiolabeled homes in on a particular organ, it is then possible to obtain pictures of that organ, using a gamma camera to detect the radioactivity that is emitted.

The amount of radiation used is very small – in many cases less than that associated with a chest X-ray. Gamma camera pictures do not give such sharp anatomical detail as IVU or CT scanning, but can provide much helpful information. There are two sorts of radionucleatide scanning used to image the kidney: static and dynamic.

Static studies

The agent injected is dimethylsuccinic acid (DMSA) that has been radiolabeled with technetium. The DMSA binds to the kidney tissues after injection into the bloodstream. About three hours after the injection, a single gamma picture of both kidneys is taken. This technique is a particular help in detecting scars on kidneys, kidneys in an unusual place (for example, in the pelvis or both on the same side) and in measuring the contribution that each kidney makes to overall kidney function. This can be very important in deciding whether a particular kidney is so diseased that it is better to remove it.

Dynamic studies

In this setting an injection of radiolabeled diethylene penta-acetic acid (DTPA) or mercaptoacyltriglycine (Mag III) is given. These agents are rapidly removed from the bloodstream by the kidney. A series of gamma camera pictures taken over the kidney and bladder area follow the excretion process as the substance is eliminated from the body. Information gained is similar to that provided by an IVU except that anatomical detail is not so precise. The technique can measure kidney function, assess blood flow to each kidney and examine whether urine drainage is being affected by some kind of obstruction.

COMPUTED TOMOGRAPHY (CT) SCANNING

CT scanning provides clear pictures of the deeper structures within the abdomen and pelvis which are less visible by ultrasound. Scans are normally undertaken after the administration of some X-ray contrast, often given by mouth to outline the bowel, and intravenously to highlight organs with a rich blood supply.

Radionucleotide scanning

a A static study of a pair of healthy human kidneys, seen from behind, shows the kidneys' blood supply as red. The blood – which was injected with a radioactive tracer before it entered the kidneys – emits gamma rays that register on this picture taken by a gamma camera.

b In another static study, one of the kidneys is healthy but the other is revealed as having a greatly reduced blood flow. Therefore the impaired kidney emits fewer gamma rays, and so the image on the picture is less bright.

CT scanning will identify the size, shape and position of the kidneys. It is an extremely useful technique for studying cysts and lesions that are suspected of being cancerous. Spread of cancer into major veins, the liver, lymph glands and the lungs can also be detected this way.

The technique allows cross-sectional reconstruction of radiographic images, which give a clear picture of the major organs of the body – as if a slice has been taken. To produce the CT scan, the patient lies in a large cylindrical structure surrounded by X-ray apparatus and computers. The procedure takes about half an hour to an hour, during which time the patient is asked to lie still. Numerous X-ray images are taken, stored and then collated by computer to produce the series of cross-sectional images.

RENAL ANGIOGRAPHY

Another method using an X-ray contrast material injected into the body, this technique focuses on the blood vessels. Renal angiography is undertaken to show the precise blood supply to the kidney and to look for abnormalities in the blood vessels themselves – for example, inflammatory conditions of the blood vessels such as polyarteritis.

The technique also shows up abnormal arteries, and new blood vessels that supply a tumour. Angiography may also be undertaken to investigate possible causes of blood in the urine (known as haematuria).

How does it work?

X-ray contrast material is injected rapidly and under high pressure into a major blood vessel. Very rapid sequence X-rays are taken over the area of interest, as the X-ray contrast arrives at the organ being studied. The X-ray contrast can be injected into a vein to obtain a picture of the venous drainage of an organ (a venogram) or intra-arterially to obtain a picture of the arterial blood supply.

MAGNETIC RESONANCE IMAGING (MRI)

MRI builds up pictures of the tissues by virtue of different energies released by different organs when exposed to an intermittent but very strong magnetic field. The technique is painless and does not expose patients to any hazardous radiation.

MRI is of particular value in producing images of soft tissues that cannot be differentiated well by X-rays, and can provide images of a similar or better quality than CT without irradiation.

As with CT imaging, the patient has to lie within a confining cylindrical structure surrounded by powerful magnets that make a loud clicking noise as the magnetic field is turned on and off. The information is stored and converted by computer into two-dimensional cross-sectional images of the body.

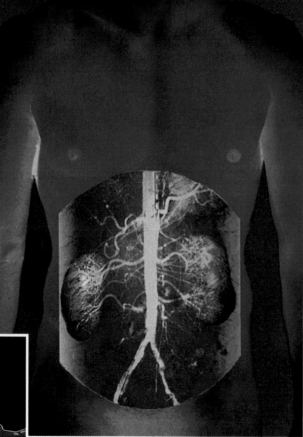

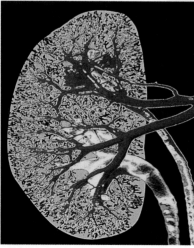

Angiograms of the blood supply to the kidneys
Above: a coloured angiogram shows as yellow the arteries supplying blood to the kidneys. The arteries branch off the abdominal aorta, which runs down the two kidneys. Left: the interior of a kidney is explored in more detail by this angiogram. Here the renal arterial system is coloured purple. Waste products pass to the bladder through the ureter, shown as yellow.

Investigations

Advances in technology have lead to the advent of 'keyhole' or minimal-access surgery, making it possible to visualise the inside of the body in great detail – and to perform operations – without having to make large incisions to gain access.

KIDNEY BIOPSY

The ability to remove a tiny piece of kidney under local anaesthetic with a needle has revolutionised the understanding and management of kidney disease. Prior to the 1960s, tissue could usually only be obtained from a kidney after the death of the patient, by which time the information to hand was severely limited because the organ was being examined at the end rather than the beginning of its disease process and much scarring would be present.

What is it used for?

Kidney biopsy has enabled a wide range of kidney diseases to be accurately classified and correlated with investigations and responses to treatment. It is now an integral part of the investigations of many kidney conditions. Diseases and disorders such as glomerulonephritis, vasculitis, amyloidosis and diabetes mellitus, plus drug toxicities, can be diagnosed from a kidney biopsy.

A biopsy will provide valuable information as to the likely outcome of a complaint – for example, whether the patient will end up needing kidney dialysis or a transplant. It may also indicate treatable diseases so that appropriate treatment can be prescribed and, equally importantly, inappropriate and potentially dangerous treatment avoided. Furthermore, following a kidney transplant the kidney may be biopsied in cases where rejection is suspected.

How does it work?

A small core of kidney tissue – about half the size of a matchstick – is removed. Sometimes it is necessary to take two or even three cores to obtain a full examination of the specimen. Diseases for which a biopsy is indicated will affect both kidneys symmetrically so that a biopsy only

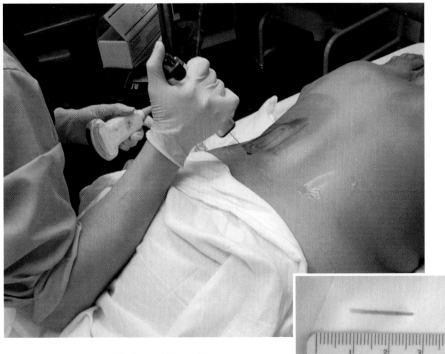

Having a kidney biopsy
The patient is asked to lie face down on a firm bed or couch and a local anaesthetic is administered. The kidney having been located using an ultrasound probe, a needle is introduced into the kidney through the patient's back. The needle removes a tiny core of kidney tissue (shown inset right at real size).

needs to be carried out on one kidney – usually on the left where the liver is not in the way. Once suitable pieces of tissue have been obtained, they are sent to the laboratory where they will be cut into very thin sections, stained and examined under a microscope.

Are there any adverse effects?

Risks associated with a kidney biopsy, if carried out by an experienced operator under ultrasound control, are very small. The risk of a bleed requiring blood transfusion is about 1 in 50–100 and the risk of a kidney tear or a deep penetration requiring removal of that kidney is less than 1 in 500.

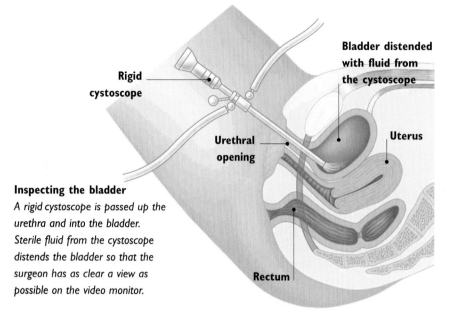

Inspecting the bladder
A rigid cystoscope is passed up the urethra and into the bladder. Sterile fluid from the cystoscope distends the bladder so that the surgeon has as clear a view as possible on the video monitor.

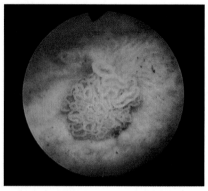

Inside the bladder
A cancerous tumour on the wall of a bladder as viewed through a cystoscope. Using the cystoscope, a biopsy specimen can be taken.

CYSTOURETHROSCOPY

This involves inspecting the urethra and bladder by passing a cystoscope (a type of telescope) up the urethra. Sterile fluid is passed through the cystoscope in order to stretch the bladder so that every fold and corner can be seen. The cystoscope also transmits light into the bladder and the image is transmitted onto a video display screen by a system of lenses, cameras and fibreoptic cables. The operator can move the cystoscope around to get a complete picture of the inside of the bladder and urethra. There are two basic designs of cystoscope:

• **Flexible cystoscope** An operator can manipulate the flexible tip of this telescope in order to see in different directions. It is narrow and has the advantage that it can be used without the need for a general anaesthetic. The disadvantage is that it is not possible to perform complex operations through a flexible cystoscope.

• **Rigid cystoscope** This is a rigid telescope and is generally used with the patient under a general anaesthetic. Again, it passes light into the bladder, and has an inflow and outflow channel for fluid. The fluid keeps the bladder distended and flushes out any debris or blood, so that a good view is maintained. The main advantage of this type of cystoscope is that fine instruments can be passed up it in order to perform surgery

inside the bladder and urethra without the need to cut open the bladder. Recovery from such operations is much quicker than from traditional 'open' surgery. The most common uses of this instrument are to take biopsies of the bladder, to crush up bladder stones (see page 118) and to relieve an obstruction in men whose prostate is enlarged (see page 130).

URETEROSCOPY

This is an inspection of the interior of a ureter (the tube that runs from a kidney down into the bladder) with a ureteroscope – a long flexible telescope similar to a cystoscope. The procedure takes place with the patient under a general anaesthetic. The ureteroscope is passed through the urethra and bladder, then up the ureter. A fibreoptic light cable, camera and a monitor enable the surgeon to see inside the ureter. Often the surgeon is looking for a stone stuck in the lower part of the ureter.

Long, fine instruments can be threaded up the ureteroscope to grab a stone and pull it out, or to break it down with laser energy or ultrasound, allowing the resulting grit to pass out of the body (see page 119).

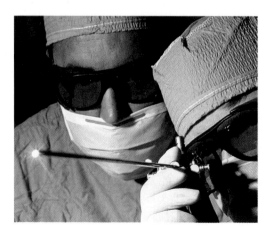

Gaining access
An instrument such as this laser device can be passed up a ureteroscope and used to destroy a stone in the urinary tract.

CURRENT TREATMENTS

Developments in modern medicine have advanced considerably in recent years, and now patients are able to enjoy partial if not full recovery from a host of conditions that were previously untreatable. For non-threatening complaints, such as incontinence and renal or urological infections, there are a number of non-pharmacological aids as well as a reliable battery of drugs and therapies. And progress in surgical methods has led to a host of solutions for treating troublesome ailments such as kidney stones, prostate problems and kidney failure.

Drugs for renal and urological problems

Many conditions affecting the kidneys and urinary tract – infections, incontinence and hypertension – can be both uncomfortable and inconvenient. Thankfully a large number of them may be treated successfully without the need for surgery.

ANTIBIOTICS FOR INFECTIONS

Widely used in the treatment of viral, fungal and bacterial infections of the kidneys and urinary tract, the majority of antibiotics are condition-specific and must be prescribed by a doctor.

Antifungals

The fungal infection vaginal candidiasis (thrush) can make urination very painful. This condition, caused by the yeast-like fungus Candida albicans, can be treated by inserting antifungal pessaries or cream high into the vagina. It may well recur if a course of treatment is not completed or if there are predisposing factors such as other antibiotics being taken, use of oral contraceptives, pregnancy or diabetes mellitus. A partner may be a source of re-infection and, if he or she also has symptoms, should be treated at the same time.

- **Imidazole drugs** – notably clotrimazole (Canesten), econazole (Ecostatin, Gyno-prevaryl) and miconazole (Gyno-daktarin) – are effective in short courses of 3 to 14 days according to the preparation used.

Divide and conquer
A Candida albicans cell is about to divide into two. Candidiasis affects the moist mucous membranes of the vagina and surrounding area; symptoms can include a burning sensation when urine is being passed.

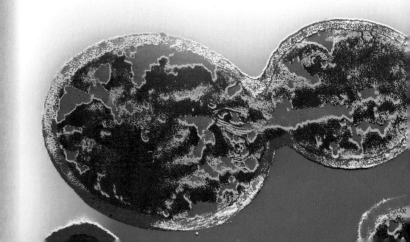

- Single-dose preparations are also available.
- Oral treatment with fluconazole (Diflucan-one) is available over the counter as a once-only capsule.

Antivirals

Antiviral drugs may be used in the treatment of initial and recurrent genital herpes simplex virus infections. They have a beneficial effect, generally giving relief from pain and other symptoms.

- Aciclovir cream (Zovirax) is used for treatment of initial and recurrent labial and genital herpes simplex infections. Use should begin as early as possible.
- Famciclovir (Famvir) and Valaciclovir (Valtrex) are suitable for vaginal infections. Available as tablets to be taken by mouth.

Antibacterials

Antibacterial drugs are effective in the treatment of many urological conditions, especially bacterial infections of the lower urinary tract, the prostate gland in men and of the kidneys.

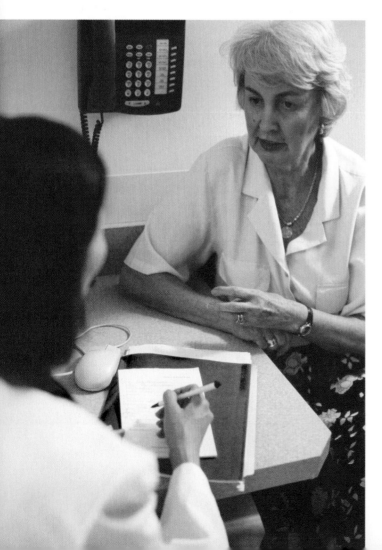

- Trimethoprim, Nitrofurantoin, Amoxycillin or Cephalexin is taken for 3 days or so for lower urinary tract infections.
- Ciprofloxacin or Trimethoprim is available as a 28-day course for prostate infections such as prostatitis.
- Ciprofloxacin or Norfloxacin can be taken for acute infections of the kidney (pyelonephritis).
- Doxycycline or Azithromycin can be used for urethral bacterial infections, commonly caused by Chlamydia trachomatis or Trichomonas vaginalis.
- Ofloxacin and Metronidazole can be taken over at least 14 days for pelvic inflammatory disease.

DRUGS FOR INCONTINENCE

The drugs available that can help combat incontinence are those that will relax or stimulate the bladder muscle or the urethral sphincter, as need be. When loss of bladder control is due to excessive contractions of the bladder muscle, a drug that reduces overactive bladder contractions may be used. In cases where the problem is an underactive bladder muscle, drug treatment will focus on stimulating contractions in this muscle. If overflow incontinence results from excessive urethral sphincter contractions, drugs that relax the urethral sphincter are available. There are also drugs to increase sphincter closure, which help with cases of stress incontinence.

Anticholinergics

An anticholinergic will relax the bladder smooth muscle, and so help to suppress involuntary bladder contractions, thereby lessening the frequency – and urgency – of the need to pass urine. Various anticholinergic drugs are available, but two of the most popular are Oxybutinin and Tolterodine.

- Oxybutinin blocks contractions of the bladder by relaxing the bladder muscle. It is generally taken several times a day, as an immediate release drug.
- Tolterodine is specifically used for an overactive bladder, It has fewer side effects than Oxybutinin.

Anticholinergic agents may cause drowsiness and blurred vision. They should be used cautiously by frail, elderly patients, who are more susceptible to adverse effects.

Discussing a drug prescription with the GP
There are drug-based treatments available for many kidney and urinary tract disorders, but the pros and cons of drug treatment in comparison with other medical and surgical alternatives should always be considered before a decision is made.

Do NSAIDs cause kidney damage?

There is substantial evidence from experimental and clinical studies that NSAIDs (nonsteroidal anti-inflammatory drugs) have a variety of effects on the kidneys. The most common renal disorder associated with NSAIDs is acute – largely reversible – failure, due to the inhibition of substances called prostaglandins, which normally cause dilation of the renal artery and encourage blood flow through the kidney. Inhibition can lead to acute renal failure in patients with specific risk factors, such as old age, hypertension, accompanying use of diuretics or aspirin, pre-existing renal failure, or diabetes. The chronic effects of NSAIDs on the kidney are less well documented than the acute effects. However, chronic renal failure can occur after the prolonged use of NSAIDs, and therefore such use should be discouraged. If it is absolutely necessary, for example in people with rheumatoid arthritis, renal function should be closely monitored.

ASK THE EXPERT

Antidepressants

Tricyclic antidepressants (TCAs) help to improve urine storage by reducing the bladder's tendency to contract and increasing resistance to urine outflow.

- **Imipramine** is a tricyclic antidepressant that reduces bladder contractions through anticholinergic effects and also increases muscle tone in the urethra. It has been used with success to treat night-time bedwetting in children (over the age of six or so), as well as incontinence in adults. There are some side effects, however, including hypotension (low blood pressure) and disturbances in the heart's conduction process, especially in older people.

DIURETICS

Diuretics are drugs that increase the amount of sodium chloride (salt) and water excreted by the kidneys. They are used in the treatment of oedema (water retention), hypertension (high blood pressure), heart failure and kidney failure. Hypertension is a frequent finding in patients with either acute or chronic kidney disease. The elevation in blood pressure is often due to fluid overload secondary to salt retention.

Loop diuretics

These are so-called because they act directly on the loop of Henle within each nephron in the kidney. They include Furosemide (Frusemide), Bumetanide and Torasemide, all of which are taken orally. At maximum dosage, loop diuretics can lead to the excretion of up to 25 per cent of filtered sodium. Side effects can include disturbances in electrolyte balance, especially hypokalaemia (low blood-potassium levels).

Thiazide diuretics

They include Bendrofluazide and Hydrochlorothiazide. When given at maximum dosage, thiazides cause excretion of 3–5 per cent of filtered sodium. High doses can cause marked changes in blood potassium, uric acid, glucose and lipids.

Potassium-sparing diuretics

These lead to the excretion of 1–2 per cent of filtered sodium. They include Amiloride, Spironolactone and Triamterene. Treatment with thiazide or loop diuretics often leads to potassium deficiency. Potassium-sparing diuretics are primarily used in combination with a loop or thiazide diuretic, either to diminish the degree of potassium loss, or to increase net diuresis in patients with unresponsive oedema.

OESTROGEN FOR INCONTINENCE

Applied as a cream or taken orally, the hormone oestrogen can be taken to help treat urge incontinence in post-menopausal women. Studies have shown that oestrogen treatment also provides significant protection against urinary tract infections.

The treatment works by encouraging colonisation of the vagina by lactobacilli (lactic-acid-producing bacteria), which keep the acidity of the vagina low and so prevent growth of bacteria that cause infections. In addition, this change of acidity is understood to discourage the development of urinary tract infections, of urinary incontinence due to involuntary contractions of the bladder muscle, and of pelvic organ prolapse.

Two relatively new delivery systems for oestrogen are a vaginal ring called Estring, and tablets to insert into the vagina, called Vagifem. Although generally well tolerated, oestrogen therapy should not be used by women who are, or may become, pregnant, or those with a history of breast, endometrial or uterine cancer.

Treatments for common types of incontinence

These are specific treatments, additional to advice on general lifestyle factors, including food and drink intake.
If possible, it's best to try exercises or behavioural therapies before resorting to treatment with drugs or surgery.

Condition	Treatment	Pros	Cons
STRESS INCONTINENCE DUE TO WEAKNESS IN THE PELVIC FLOOR MUSCLE	Exercises for pelvic floor muscle, with biofeedback	The exercises are easy to do, anytime, anywhere.	Can take a long time to see improvement; the condition may be improved rather than cured.
	SURGICAL Colposuspension for a weak bladder neck	High success rate.	Possibility of developing urge incontinence.
	Tension-free vaginal tape	Minimally invasive, with a high success rate.	Long-term success rate data is not yet available.
	Sling procedure	Successful after alternatives have been tried but failed.	Self-catheterisation may become necessary.
STRESS INCONTINENCE DUE TO WEAKNESS IN THE SPHINCTER MUSCLES	**DRUGS** Drugs to help tighten the sphincter muscles	Helps to relieve mild stress incontinence.	As with all drugs, there may be side effects.
	SURGICAL Artificial sphincter cuff	High success rate.	Cuff sometimes regarded as too artificial.
URGE INCONTINENCE DUE TO INVOLUNTARY CONTRACTIONS OF THE BLADDER MUSCLE	Bladder training	Increases the time between attacks of urgency to urinate.	Condition may be improved but not cured.
	Exercises to strengthen the pelvic muscle	Helps the patient resist an urge to urinate until a toilet can be reached.	Condition may be improved but not cured.
	Behavioural therapy/ biofeedback	Enables the patient to recognise and hold back contractions.	Condition may be improved but not cured.
	DRUGS Anticholinergic drugs	Can be effective.	Success varies from patient to patient; patients may suffer side effects.
	Oestrogen treatment	Can be effective.	Success varies from patient to patient; patients may suffer side effects.
	SURGICAL Clam cystoplasty	Possibility of improved quality of life for patients with severely overactive bladders.	Possibility of major side effects.
	Removal of the bladder	Relief from incontinence caused by an overactive bladder.	Permanent loss of bladder makes urinary diversion surgery (see page 129) and a urine-collecting bag necessary.
OVERFLOW INCONTINENCE DUE TO AN ENLARGED PROSTATE GLAND	**SURGICAL** Transurethral resection of the prostate (TURP)	High success rate.	Some sexual function may be lost; side effects may include retrograde ejaculation.
	Removal of the prostate gland	Alternative if TURP is not enough to solve the problem.	Likelihood of some loss of sexual function; possibility of incontinence.

Medical solutions

As well as drug therapy there are a number of other therapies that help to improve bladder dysfunction. Most are supervised by continence advisors or physiotherapists. All require a patient to be highly motivated and to devote enough time to them to gain the full benefits.

BLADDER TRAINING

This is a method of improving the symptoms caused by an overactive 'unstable' bladder. In this disorder, the bladder is oversensitive and sends messages to the brain that it is full and needs to be emptied urgently, when it is in fact not full at all.

To bring the problem under control, it is necessary to learn to stretch the bladder. This is achieved by holding on for as long as possible when there is the urge to pass urine. This difficult task becomes easier with time. Patients should aim to reduce the frequency with which they pass urine to 5 or 6 times in 24 hours, whilst drinking 1.5 to 2 litres (2½ to 3½ pints) a day. This is often accompanied by the use of anticholinergic drugs to relax the bladder. Doctors have found that three out of four patients who undertake bladder training experience a significant improvement in their symptoms.

Help with bladder training
A patient at a hospital outpatients department receives advice on how the bladder works and how best to monitor fluid intake and urine output, as part of her bladder training therapy.

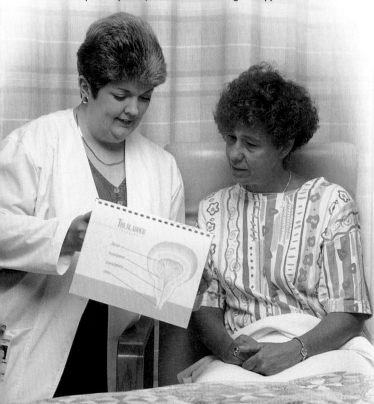

BEHAVIOURAL THERAPY

This method aims to overcome bladder symptoms by demonstrating the presence of abnormal bladder contractions, with the use of a pressure monitor linked up to a light or a bell, and then teaching the patient to hold back these contractions. This is known as biofeedback. It helps by teaching more about the abnormality that is causing the symptoms and by providing instant visual feedback on how well the patient is controlling them. In research trials, six out of ten patients reported improvement. However, biofeedback is unlikely to completely cure the symptoms on its own, and requires both patient and therapist to be motivated and persistent.

The same technique of biofeedback can be used as a way of teaching effective pelvic floor contractions as part of pelvic floor physiotherapy. It involves using either a mechanical device placed inside the vagina, called a perineometer, or an electrical sensor to detect the strength of pelvic floor contractions. Using this read-out over a period of time, it is possible to train the pelvic floor muscles to contract more efficiently.

LIFESTYLE ADVICE

Often, bladder symptoms can be improved by making a few simple lifestyle changes. A chart noting how much urine is passed and how often will allow a doctor or specialist nurse to pinpoint changes that will help.

Drinking more than 1.5 to 2 litres (2½ to 3½ pints) a day can make an overactive bladder worse. Cutting down on drinks in the evening and before bed will reduce unwanted night-time trips to the toilet or episodes of leakage. Eliminating bladder stimulants such as coffee, tea, cola and alcohol from the diet will make the bladder less 'unstable'. A doctor may suggest to a patient that the bladder be emptied regularly every 1–2 hours even if there is not felt to be a need, in order to avoid leaking.

Advice on how best to lose weight and/or stop smoking is often offered. Being overweight exerts extra pressure on the bladder, causing it to leak more often. Smoking causes more frequent coughing, which also

Incontinence aids for women

a Vaginal cones are a way of building up pelvic floor muscle strength. They consist of four or five different weights that can be placed inside a plastic cone. A cone plus the lightest weight is inserted into the vagina and then held in place by squeezing the pelvic muscles for 20 minutes or so, daily. When this becomes easy, the user moves to the next weight up. By the time the heaviest cone is in use, the pelvic floor muscles should be much stronger.

b There are bladder neck supports available that can be used via either the vagina or (as shown here) the urethra. By supporting the bladder neck, the device reduces accidental urine leakage. It can be used all day, or just during exercise, when the chances of leakage are greatest.

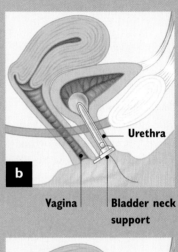

Urethra

b

Vagina | Bladder neck support

c Devices that block off the exit to the urethra act like a plug. They take the form of a foam cap that is stuck onto the urethral opening with gel (as shown here) or of devices that fit up inside the urethra to plug it off.

Rectum

Bladder

Cone in vagina

Urethra

a

Pelvic floor muscles

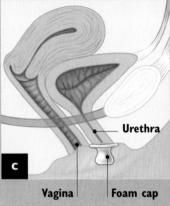

Urethra

c

Vagina | Foam cap

squeezes the bladder. Anyone considering surgical treatment for incontinence should certainly try to lose any extra weight and stop smoking (if applicable); this will make the operation safer and increase the chances of long-term success.

PELVIC FLOOR PHYSIOTHERAPY

This is usually the first line of treatment for patients whose incontinence is related to weakness in the pelvic floor muscles. The pelvic floor plays a key role in helping to hold the bladder in its correct position so that it can function normally. Women are much more susceptible to pelvic floor weakness than men, because of the effects of pregnancy and childbirth. Weakness can lead to leaking urine when coughing, sneezing or exercising.

A physiotherapist will tailor pelvic floor exercise techniques to individual need. The first step is to be taught where the pelvic floor muscles are, and how to contract them voluntarily if the patient does not already

know how to do this. The physiotherapist's fingers, or a pressure-measuring device called a perineometer, can gauge the strength of a pelvic floor contraction. The patient is then given a series of exercises to perform at home; there are check-ups with the physiotherapist to monitor progress.

Improvement is gradual, over a period of time. Exercisers therefore need to be motivated and to devote sufficient time to this treatment to get the maximum benefit out of it.

NEUROMODULATION

This is a new treatment for incontinence caused by an overactive bladder. It involves planting an electrical pulse generator inside the body to send electrical impulses to the nerves supplying the bladder; these impulses inhibit bladder overactivity. At present this treatment tends to be prescribed for patients who have not been satisfactorily treated by other more established treatments.

ANTI-INCONTINENCE DEVICES

Various devices are available to help control incontinence. These can be useful for patients who are not fit enough for surgery or who don't wish to have an operation. They are also useful for patients who experience problems only sometimes, such as when doing strenuous exercise.

Absorbent products

Modern incontinence pads – specially designed for men and women suffering from urinary incontinence – are discreet, highly absorbent and comfortable even when wet. The perceived social stigma of urinary incontinence means that often patients are slow to seek help, and 'make do' with sanitary towels or tissue paper. It is far better to talk to a continence adviser and find out which products best suit each case.

Incontinence pads should not be used as an alternative to a more effective medical solution. Rather, they should be seen as a temporary measure, while tests are underway, or the full benefits of treatment are being awaited.

Penile clamps

For men who are incontinent, usually as a result of prostate gland surgery, a device called a penile clamp is available. This squeezes the shaft of the penis and so closes off the urethra running along the centre of it. When it is convenient to empty the bladder, the clamp is released and the bladder allowed to drain.

CATHETERS

The purpose of a urinary catheter is to ensure that the bladder is completely drained. A catheter is usually necessary either when there is a physical obstruction preventing adequate drainage, or the bladder muscle is too weak to effectively empty the bladder. The reason why it is so important to keep the bladder properly drained is because stagnant urine sitting in the bladder will become infected. In addition, urine that can't be drained from the body could flow towards the kidneys, potentially causing damage and scarring.

Another reason for inserting a catheter is to 'rest' the bladder. This is often done after an operation or following a bladder injury repair, when the patient doesn't want the bladder to fill up and exert pressure on the repair stitches.

Catheters can be inserted through the urethra (a urethral catheter), or through the skin in front of the bladder at approximately the level of the pubic hairline (a suprapubic catheter). They are made in a variety of sizes and in different materials.

Clean intermittent self catheterisation (CISC) is usually the best option for patients needing to use a catheter in the long-term as well as in the short-term. The drawback with a suprapubic catheter is that it is permanently in place; an indwelling urethral catheter becomes uncomfortable if left in place for any length of time.

Catheters for men and women

a Clean intermittent self catheterisation (CISC) involves passing a fine, sterile catheter into the bladder to drain it. The catheter is then removed. The procedure needs to be repeated approximately every 4 hours, depending on fluid intake. The bladder should never be allowed to hold more than 500ml (just under 1 pint); more than this would overstretch the muscle fibres and potentially cause lasting damage.

b A suprapubic catheter designed for long-term use is inserted by a surgeon with the patient under local or general anaesthetic. It is replaced every three months or so. The urine is either allowed to drain continuously into a bag attached to the leg or is let out intermittently by means of a valve.

A suprapubic catheter is best for those who are for some reason unable to cope with the CISC procedure.

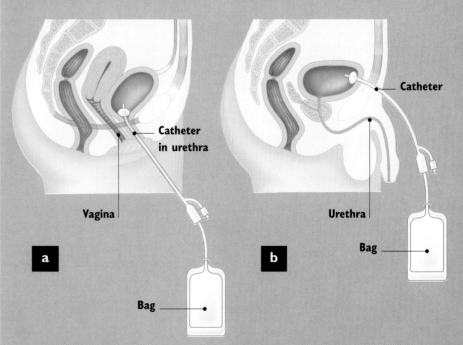

a — Vagina | Catheter in urethra | Bag

b — Urethra | Catheter | Bag

Kidney dialysis

Dialysis is a process of artificially purifying the blood to remove the toxins that accumulate after kidney failure. Dialysis also allows the removal of excess fluid and the maintenance of safe levels of electrolytes such as potassium.

HOW DIALYSIS WORKS

In the dialysis process, blood loaded with toxins is separated from dialysis fluid by just a semi-permeable membrane. Waste products, salts and extra fluids move from the blood, across the membrane and into the dialysis fluid, by the processes of diffusion and filtration.

Dialysis can either take place outside the body with the aid of a dialysis machine (this is haemodialysis, HD) or inside the body, using the natural membrane lining the abdominal cavity (peritoneal dialysis, PD).

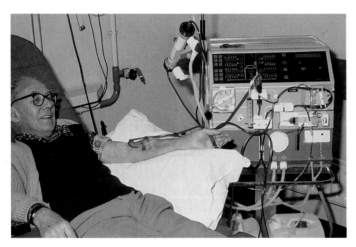

WHO NEEDS DIALYSIS?

Dialysis treatment protects from the life-threatening complications of uraemia (see page 154), such as fluid retention and high blood potassium levels. It may be required for any patient with kidney failure, either acute or chronic (see page 145).

Whether or not dialysis is required and the timing of treatment is a matter of clinical judgement, which must take into account the level of toxins in the blood, the amount of excess fluid in the patient and the likelihood of imminent recovery of kidney function. Urgent treatment may be required if, for example, high potassium levels cause irritation of the heart or fluid accumulates in the lungs causing breathing difficulties. In patients with acute kidney failure, dialysis is usually only needed temporarily, until kidney function recovers. Individuals with chronic kidney failure require long-term treatment that can only be discontinued if they receive a kidney transplant.

Women on dialysis are advised not to conceive, since a pregnancy will most likely lead to miscarriage or a very premature baby. The dialysis process means that many women can't conceive anyway; those who can are advised to use effective birth control (but not the contraceptive pill). Men on dialysis can father children.

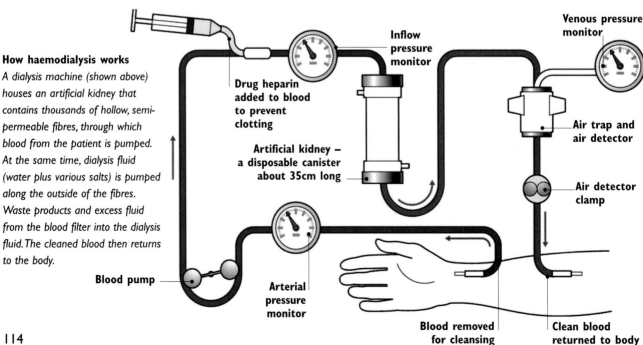

How haemodialysis works
A dialysis machine (shown above) houses an artificial kidney that contains thousands of hollow, semi-permeable fibres, through which blood from the patient is pumped. At the same time, dialysis fluid (water plus various salts) is pumped along the outside of the fibres. Waste products and excess fluid from the blood filter into the dialysis fluid. The cleaned blood then returns to the body.

Blood pump

Drug heparin added to blood to prevent clotting

Artificial kidney – a disposable canister about 35cm long

Arterial pressure monitor

Inflow pressure monitor

Venous pressure monitor

Air trap and air detector

Air detector clamp

Blood removed for cleansing

Clean blood returned to body

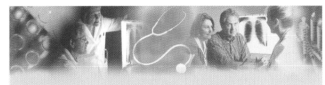

Milestones
IN MEDICINE

The great breakthrough in developing a human dialysis machine came in the early 1940s, when a Dutch medical researcher, Willem J. Kolff, developed his 'Kolff artificial kidney'. Kolff later sent copies of this machine to the UK, Canada and the USA, but uptake and enthusiasm was very limited until the early 1960s. The change came after the 'Scribner shunt' was invented in Seattle in 1960; this made access to the patient's bloodstream considerably easier, and for the first time repeated dialysis for patients with chronic kidney failure became a practical possibility.

HAEMODIALYSIS – OUTSIDE THE BODY

In haemodialysis, blood purification takes place outside the body in an 'artificial kidney'. Blood leaves the patient's body, passes through the dialysis machine that contains the artificial kidney and then returns into the patient's body. Haemodialysis has been in common use since the 1960s.

How blood leaves and enters the body

Access to the patient's circulation is gained through the surgical construction of an artificial connection – an arteriovenous fistula – between an artery and a vein in the arm or wrist. About 8 weeks after the operation to create this fistula, two needles can be inserted into vessels in the fistula, so blood can be removed for dialysis at the necessary flow rate of 300ml per minute, then returned.

Alternatively, a pair of tubes can be inserted into large veins in the neck or groin. This is for patients who need dialysis at once and so can't wait for a fistula to heal.

When and where haemodialysis takes place

Most patients on haemodialysis require about four hours treatment three times a week, depending the level of residual kidney function and their body build. In the past, some patients have had a dialysis machine in their home, but the increasing availability of dialysis units in the community has made this unnecessary, and most patients do not need to travel far to receive their treatment.

PERITONEAL DIALYSIS – INSIDE THE BODY

Peritoneal dialysis (PD) is an alternative to haemodialysis for patients with chronic kidney failure. In PD, dialysis is a continuous process, during which a patient can move around and carry on with life as normal. There is usually no dialysis machine – instead, dialysis takes place inside the patient's abdomen. PD has been available since the 1980s.

When the peritoneal cavity – normally empty – is filled with dialysis fluid, toxins diffuse out of the bloodstream, across the semi-permeable membrane that lines the cavity, and into the dialysis fluid. Several times a day the patient must drain the dialysis fluid from the abdomen through a specially fitted catheter, and replace it with fresh fluid.

When and where dialysis fluids are exchanged

Generally, a patient exchanges fluids after waking, at lunchtime, in early evening and before bed, each exchange taking about 30 minutes. Exchanges must take place in a clean environment, usually a dedicated area in a patient's home, or a room at work. The exchange process can be performed by a machine that enables exchanges to take place while the patient is asleep at night.

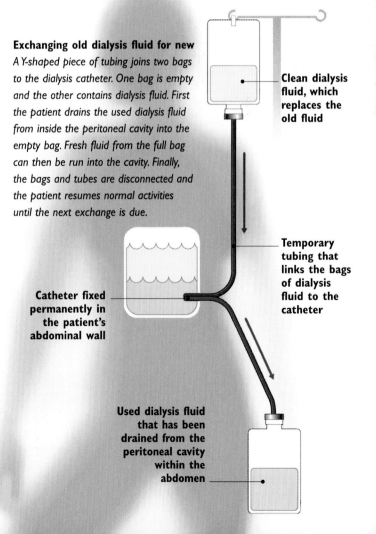

Exchanging old dialysis fluid for new
A Y-shaped piece of tubing joins two bags to the dialysis catheter. One bag is empty and the other contains dialysis fluid. First the patient drains the used dialysis fluid from inside the peritoneal cavity into the empty bag. Fresh fluid from the full bag can then be run into the cavity. Finally, the bags and tubes are disconnected and the patient resumes normal activities until the next exchange is due.

Clean dialysis fluid, which replaces the old fluid

Temporary tubing that links the bags of dialysis fluid to the catheter

Catheter fixed permanently in the patient's abdominal wall

Used dialysis fluid that has been drained from the peritoneal cavity within the abdomen

Dialysis on holiday

One of the major drawbacks of dialysis is that patients must be in a fixed location two or three times a week, or have daily access to dialysis fluid. This used to make travelling difficult for patients with kidney disorders, but things are improving.

Most people need a break from time to time, and kidney patients and their carers are no exception. For anyone needing dialysis, travel requires planning, but it is getting easier year by year. Today dialysis is no obstacle to taking a holiday. There are few constraints on holiday type or destination: haemodialysis (HD) patients can book into other units, and peritoneal dialysis (PD) patients can have supplies delivered around the world. The key to a successful trip is planning. It can take several months to finalise arrangements, so late bookings are difficult. Patients should ask their renal unit for advice.

HAEMODIALYSIS PATIENTS – FINDING A UNIT

When deciding where to go on holiday, patients need to be flexible and do some research, as it may take time to find an HD unit available for the dates and hours required.

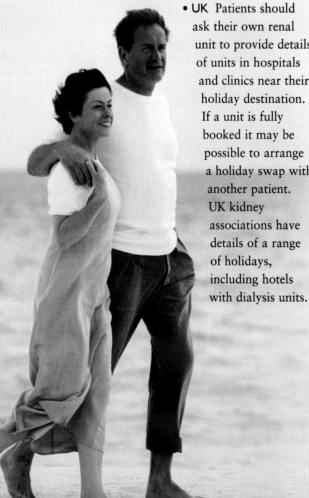

- **UK** Patients should ask their own renal unit to provide details of units in hospitals and clinics near their holiday destination. If a unit is fully booked it may be possible to arrange a holiday swap with another patient. UK kidney associations have details of a range of holidays, including hotels with dialysis units.

SPECIAL ARRANGEMENTS CHECKLIST

- **Vaccinations** All immunisations (including hepatitis B) must be up to date. If vaccinations for particular countries are required, patients should check with their renal unit because some are not recommended for kidney patients.
- **Medications** Patients must carry a letter from their GP listing their medication when passing through customs. If medication needs to be kept cool, patients should carry a soft cool-bag with ice packs, and pre-arrange for the airline to store it in a fridge during the flight. Take care to carry medicines in hand luggage in case of delays.
- **Dietary requirements** All airlines and cruise ships, and many hotels, cater for special diets (such as salt-free, low protein), but the meals must be requested in advance. Self-catering holidays allow greater flexibility, although patients should talk to their dietitian about foods to avoid while away.
- **Assistance at airports** Patients who tire easily or have problems with mobility can ask their travel agent to pre-book a buggy to travel through the airport, and arrange assistance getting on and off the plane. If necessary, oxygen can be arranged during the flight, although some airlines may charge a substantial fee.

- **Abroad** There is a wealth of information available on the internet. Stories from individual patients can inspire adventurous trips, and directories list where dialysis units can be found. Patients can contact units directly (for information, to check availability or to reserve a session) or use a specialist travel agent.

Every unit will require copies of the following before they are able to confirm a patient's booking: a full set of blood tests; dialysis details and flow sheet; medications taken; a doctor's letter with medical history; a chest X-ray and an ECG. The patient's own renal unit will supply these.

PERITONEAL DIALYSIS PATIENTS

PD patients can holiday just about anywhere, as dialysis fluid can be delivered to a wide range of destinations. This is arranged through the fluid supply company or the patient's own renal unit. They will need destination contact details and holiday dates. It is important to plan in advance – when travelling abroad the notice required can be up to four months, although the average is two.

When patients are choosing accommodation they must check it is possible to have PD supplies delivered a few days before their arrival, and that delivery and storage facilities are available.

There are a number of practical issues for PD patients to bear in mind. Firstly, it is important that travel plans be discussed with a renal nurse, so a suitable exchange plan can be devised. Exchanges must be carried out in a clean, safe environment. It's better to delay an exchange rather than carry it out in an unhygienic or cramped area. At airports, exchanges can be carried out in the medical room or St John's Ambulance treatment room.

Before travelling, patients should ask for advice on disposing of the waste: prior arrangements need to be made with the nearest hospital or surgery. Waste should never be left behind as it is considered a health hazard.

COST

Patients should not book their holiday until they have holiday insurance which covers pre-existing medical conditions. Insurance companies may require a letter from the patient's renal unit confirming they are fit to travel.

If travelling to an EU country, patients should complete an E111 form available from post offices. EU countries have reciprocal arrangements with the UK for dialysis. The E111 form entitles the holder to free or subsidised treatment in state-run clinics or hospitals. However, do check with individual dialysis units before booking the holiday. The UK also has reciprocal arrangements with Australia and New Zealand, but dialysis must be paid for in the USA.

HOLIDAY PRECAUTIONS

- **Food and drink** Patients should watch what they eat and drink while abroad. They should drink bottled or boiled water. Salads, ice cubes and ice cream from street stalls should be avoided.

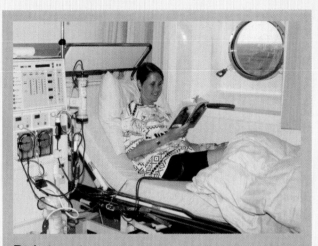

Dialysis cruises

Specialist holidays catering for the needs of dialysis patients, including dialysis cruises, have become extremely popular. The ships have a dialysis unit and nephrology staff on board. They support between 10 and 12 dialysis patients, so it is important to book ahead. The itinerary is scheduled around dialysis treatments so patients will not miss out on planned tours or activities. When the ship is in port treatments are scheduled early in the morning or at the end of the day to allow patients the maximum amount of time off the ship. Staff ensure that patients receive the same number of treatments as they would at home.

- **Swimming** Before travelling, patients should check with their renal unit for advice on swimming and other sports.
- **Sun protection** A high factor sunscreen should be used, and overexposure to the sun avoided. This is particularly important for transplant patients.
- **First aid kit** In addition to a standard first aid kit, patients should take gauze and tape in case of bleeding at their exit site and some antibacterial soap to clean their exit site prior to dialysis.
- **Emergencies** Patients should ensure they have emergency contact numbers with them, including a medical contact at their destination, numbers of their UK renal unit, travel agent and insurance company. They should wear a medical alert tag and carry an instruction sheet listing their condition and medicines, in more than one language.

Surgical solutions

There is a vast range of operations that can be performed on the kidneys and urinary tract. Many involve the trusted techniques of open surgery, but laparoscopic surgery has revolutionised treatment in this field.

Surgery is the solution only when a condition cannot be treated effectively in any other way. Surgery on the kidneys, bladder or urinary tract may be performed:
• to rid the system of painful kidney or bladder stones;
• to alleviate incontinence and pain when passing urine;
• to replace failed kidneys with one that functions;
• to combat cancer.
Since the effects of surgery are largely irreversible, it is essential that patient and surgeon discuss in advance the various surgical solutions, taking the benefits, the likelihood of success, and side effects into account.

LAPAROSCOPIC SURGERY
With the patient under a general anaesthetic, carbon dioxide gas is used to distend the abdominal cavity and a laparoscope (a type of endoscope) is inserted through a cut in the navel. Long, slender instruments are then introduced through additional incisions. The surgeon manoeuvres them while looking at a monitor showing the view inside the abdomen. This allows the surgeon:
• to explore the organs within the abdomen;
• to take samples for further examination in a laboratory;
• to perform surgery that would otherwise have required a large incision to gain access to the operation site.
The advantages over 'open' surgery are less pain for the patient and a more rapid return to normal life. But there is a small risk that instruments could accidentally damage the bladder, bowel or blood vessels.

OPEN SURGERY
Traditional open surgery remains the most appropriate choice in many cases, as when a cancerous kidney is removed (see page 128) and sometimes the only choice, as in a kidney transplant (see page 122). Even when a minimally invasive operation is an option, open surgery may still be preferred if the surgeon is best skilled in traditional techniques. An operation performed with 'keyhole' surgery does not always have a better outcome, with better long-term results or fewer complications.

Removing stones

Bladder stone removal was one of the few successful operations before the advent of modern anaesthesia and hygiene. Today there are various ways to find and extract stones from the bladder, kidneys or urinary tract.

SURGERY INVOLVING A CYSTOSCOPE
The modern laparoscopic treatment for bladder stones involves passing a cystoscope (a type of endoscope that is inserted via the urethra) into the bladder while the patient is under a general anaesthetic. The urologist begins by using the cystoscope to inspect the bladder and give any stones present in the bladder a close examination. Then a choice is made from the small armoury of devices with which these stones can be tackled.
• A lithrotrite is a modified cystoscope with stone-crushing jaws. It will crush bladder stones into fragments, which are then washed out by irrigating the bladder with a sterile solution.
• A wire basket or snare can be fed along the cystoscope – or along its sister instrument the ureteroscope, which can examine farther up the urinary tract, as far as the kidneys. The basket or snare captures a stone and pulls it out through the bladder and urethra.

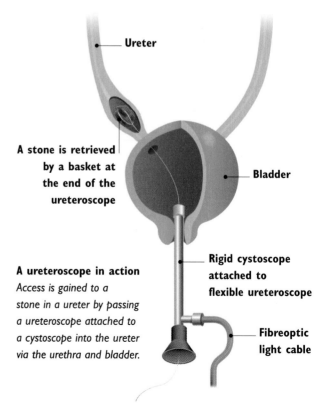

Ureter

A stone is retrieved by a basket at the end of the ureteroscope

Bladder

Rigid cystoscope attached to flexible ureteroscope

Fibreoptic light cable

A ureteroscope in action
Access is gained to a stone in a ureter by passing a ureteroscope attached to a cystoscope into the ureter via the urethra and bladder.

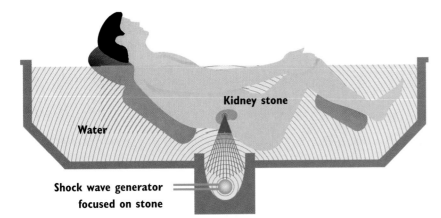

Kidney stone

Water

Shock wave generator
focused on stone

How ESWL works

ESWL uses a principle similar to a depth charge attacking a submarine: basically, a shock wave travelling through water. A machine generates a series of shock waves, which are focused on the target stone. The shock waves travel through the tissues of the body, which are mostly made of water; when they reach the stone they break it up.

- Fibres carrying laser or ultrasound energy can also be fed along these instruments and used to shatter stones stuck in one or other of the ureters that lead to the kidneys. The resulting stone fragments are small enough to travel down the urinary tract to the outside of the body. To help these fragments on their way, a double-J splint – a fine tube specially designed for the job – can be inserted into a ureter. This tube (often called a stent) is threaded up the ureter from the bladder, with the help of a cystoscope. The stent has two curly ends that keep it in place. It can be left in the ureter for several months. The presence of this foreign body causes the ureter to dilate, with the result that stone pieces that might otherwise have got stuck easily pass down to the bladder.

EXTRACORPOREAL SHOCK WAVE LITHOTRIPSY (ESWL)

Just as the techniques of minimal access surgery have revolutionised the treatment of stone disease in the bladder and ureters, so the invention of extracorporeal shock wave lithotripsy has radically improved the treatment of stones in the kidneys over the last two decades. The great advantage of ESWL over pre-existing surgical treatments is that it treats stone disease without the need to cut open the body. The risks involved and the likely duration of recovery are therefore much reduced.

Patients undergoing ESWL attend hospital as day patients, rather than having to stay in hospital overnight. Painkillers range from a general anaesthetic to a light

"EXPERIENCING EXTRACORPOREAL SHOCK WAVE LITHOTRIPSY

My doctor explained that the stone in my left kidney would be best removed by a treatment called extracorporeal shock wave lithotripsy.

On the day, I went to the outpatients department of the hospital to which I had been referred, where the urologist explained the procedure to me. I was given a dose of pethidine as a painkiller and sedative, so that I would not be made uncomfortable by the effects of the shock waves on the stone. Then I was asked to lie down on a reclining seat which was lowered into a large tub of water.

The exact position of the stone was located by two X-ray units called fluoroscopes, one on each side of me. This information was used to target the stone precisely.

The treatment consisted of a series of shock waves – several hundred as far as I could tell – over a period of about 90 minutes. Each wave was generated by an electrode or 'spark plug', which vaporised a small amount of water, creating the shock wave focused on the stone. The process wasn't painful, but seemed to take a long time and I was aware of the waves.

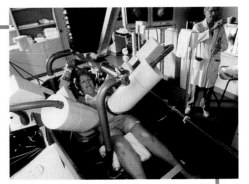

After the procedure had finished, I was advised to drink plenty of fluid to help to wash out the remaining small fragments. I was told that I would pass gritty, sand-like debris in my urine, possibly for several weeks, and that I might need to take painkillers to counteract any discomfort this might cause. I left the hospital with painkillers, which I founded I needed occasionally. "

Two ways of removing stones by percutaneous nephrolithotomy

a The jaws of a rigid endoscope clasp a kidney stone after its removal. The endoscope was introduced through a small incision in the abdomen.

b An electro-mechanical spark discharge device fragments a stone inside the kidney. The fragments are then removed via the operating sheath.

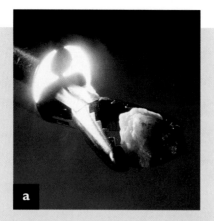

a

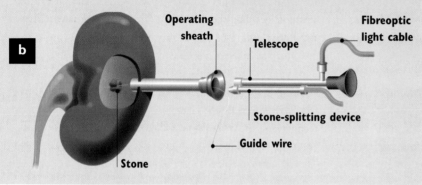

b

Operating sheath

Telescope

Fibreoptic light cable

Stone-splitting device

Guide wire

Stone

allow fine instruments to be passed into the kidney. This procedure is called a percutaneous nephrolithotomy. The rise in popularity of lithotripsy in recent years (see page 119) has greatly reduced the number of nephrolithotomies performed. But they are still the best option when:

• shock waves cannot reach a stone because a bone is in the way;
• a stone is too large to be broken up by ESWL alone;
• the stone is so large that after ESWL the amount of debris passing down the urinary tract would result in prolonged pain and obstruction.

A percutaneous nephrolithotomy

With the patient under a general anaesthetic, a long needle is passed through the skin towards the affected kidney. Either ultrasound scanning or X-rays are used to provide continuous imaging to guide the tip of the needle to the correct position.

As soon as this needle-track from the flank into the kidney has been established, it is expanded by passing a series of dilating rods through the opening. Each rod is very slightly wider than the last; by passing each in turn up the track into the kidney, a tunnel up to 1cm wide is created. Along this tunnel the urologist passes various instruments. To begin with, a nephroscope is introduced to allow the urologist to see the kidney and any stones inside it. The urologist then selects an instrument with which to destroy the stone or stones. Strong graspers for crushing, ultrasonic drills for fragmenting and lasers for shattering are among the tools available.

Larger fragments are brought out through the tunnel by grabbing them with steerable graspers or a wire basket. Smaller stone fragments and debris pass down the urinary tract towards the bladder.

After the operation, the tunnel closes up on its own. Stitches are only needed to close the small incision in the skin. Because the scar is so much smaller, recovery after a percutaneous nephrolithotomy is much quicker than after a traditional open operation.

sedative depending on the type of machine being used and the stone size. Some machines require the patient to lie in a bath of water during the procedure, while for others the patient lies on a couch. X-ray images or ultrasound are used to locate the position of the kidney stone on which shock waves will be targeted. The time needed to shatter a stone depends on its size and chemical composition. Shock waves keep on coming until the stone breaks into fragments that can pass down the urinary tract.

If multiple stones are being broken down with ESWL, a lot of pulverised debris can be expected. In this case, a double-J stent is often passed up the ureter before commencing ESWL. This causes the ureter to dilate and makes it easier for the fragments of stone to pass along the ureter, into the bladder and out of the body.

NEPHROLITHOTOMY

This is an operation in which an incision is made through the skin of the abdomen, in order to remove a stone from the kidney. A traditional open nephrolithotomy is performed through an incision about 15cm (6in) long, running just under the rib cage and curving around from back to front. Nowadays, it is more usual to create a small track from the skin into the centre of the kidney to

Surgery for stress incontinence

A variety of operations have been devised for the treatment of stress incontinence. Different operations suit different patients, depending on their symptoms, previous medical history and the results of urodynamic investigations into the causes of their stress incontinence.

The mechanisms by which urine leaks from the bladder on coughing, sneezing or exercising are varied, and it is important to establish the cause of urine leakage before deciding on surgery. Often the cause is a weak bladder neck, for which surgery is a potential solution. But in at least a tenth of cases the cause is an overactive, unstable bladder, in which case surgery to correct a weak bladder neck may make the patient's symptoms worse.

COLPOSUSPENSION

This operation offers a nine out of ten cure rate and even after ten years the cure rates are still high. The operation is performed through a 'bikini-line' incision, using laparoscopic or open surgical techniques. The surgeon places stitches around the neck of the bladder and attaches them up to a ligament on the pelvic bone. This lifts up and supports the bladder neck so it is less likely to leak. A suprapubic catheter is left in the bladder for a few days after the operation to allow the bladder to 'rest'. The benefits of the operation will last longer if lifestyle changes are made to help protect the bladder, such as eating and drinking sensibly and regularly exercising the pelvic floor.

Unfortunately, for just over a tenth of patients the operation makes the bladder muscle more unstable, leading to a frequent, urgent need to pass urine.

SLING PROCEDURES

In this operation – almost always for women – the urethra is supported by a sling made of synthetic material or a strip of muscle from the abdomen. The sling passes under the urethra, providing support in a similar way to a hammock and partially obstructing the bladder so that urine is less likely to leak out. The operation is usually performed using laparoscopic techniques.

This procedure is generally only used after other operations such as colposuspension have failed. This is because, although just over three-quarters of operations are successful, the complication rate is greater than for colposuspension. Complications can include difficulty emptying the bladder, in which case a patient must learn to perform clean intermittent self catheterisation.

TENSION-FREE VAGINAL TAPE (TVT)

Tape made of a woven artificial material is inserted in a similar way to a sling, under the urethra. This new, minimally invasive operation has quickly become popular because it is relatively easy to perform, it appears to have a high success rate, and needs only one or two nights in hospital. Immediate cure rates are similar to those for colposuspension. However, the long-term effectiveness of TVT is not yet proven.

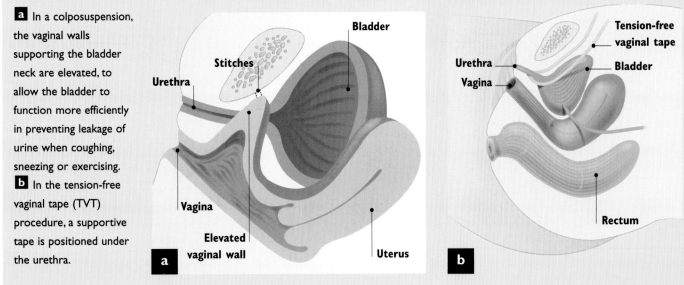

Two surgical treatments for stress incontinence

a In a colposuspension, the vaginal walls supporting the bladder neck are elevated, to allow the bladder to function more efficiently in preventing leakage of urine when coughing, sneezing or exercising. **b** In the tension-free vaginal tape (TVT) procedure, a supportive tape is positioned under the urethra.

Bladder
Stitches
Urethra
Vagina
Elevated vaginal wall
Uterus

Tension-free vaginal tape
Urethra
Vagina
Bladder
Rectum

INJECTABLE AGENTS

A technique used to combat stress incontinence in men as well as women is to inject a substance into the wall of the urethra to 'bulk it out'. This enables the bladder to form a better seal, allowing it to block the leakage of urine. Natural collagen is used, along with synthetic materials. The procedure is quick and can be done under local anaesthetic. However, multiple treatments are required, because it's hard to guess how much collagen will be needed, and because the collagen is slowly absorbed into the body, and so there must be regular top-up injections, possibly as often as every six months.

ARTIFICIAL SPHINCTER

Artificial sphincter implants are mostly used by men who have developed incontinence after a prostatectomy and in whom other treatments have failed. They have also been tried by women, but not as a first-line treatment. Artificial sphincters are wholly implanted in a patient's body.

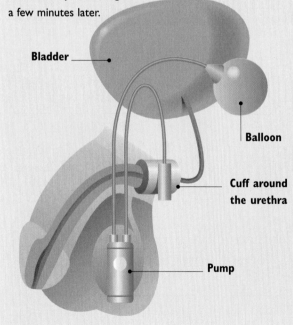

An artificial sphincter in action

The cuff, inflated with fluid, blocks off the urethra so that urine doesn't leak out. Before urinating, the patient has to squeeze the pump – implanted in the scrotum – to move fluid from the cuff to the balloon so that the cuff deflates and urine is able to drain from the bladder. The cuff automatically inflates again a few minutes later.

Bladder

Balloon

Cuff around the urethra

Pump

Kidney transplants

Kidney transplantation has come of age and is now the preferred form of treatment for patients with advanced kidney failure who would otherwise need life-long dialysis or face death.

Kidney transplantation is one of the great surgical success stories, yet there are two major problems that have still to be conquered. The first is that there are not enough kidneys available for transplant. The shortfall between the number of kidneys available for transplant and the number of patients in need of a new kidney means there is a constant waiting list. Secondly, following transplantation all patients require drugs to suppress their immune response to prevent rejection. It is the complications and side effects of these drugs that account for most of the drawbacks to kidney transplantation. However, this is becoming less of a problem as new drugs are developed and doctors become better at tailoring immunosuppression to the needs of the individual patient.

KIDNEY DONORS

Of the healthy kidneys used for transplantation, 70–80 per cent come from donors who are brainstem dead but are being maintained on a ventilator. The remaining 20–30 per cent of kidneys are from living donors; most of these are a close blood relative of the recipient.

Cadaver donors

Most kidneys used for transplants are taken from patients who have died very recently. To be considered as an organ donor, a patient must have sustained irreversible brainstem death and thus be incapable of recovery. Such patients can be maintained on a ventilator for a few days – sometimes longer – with the heart continuing to beat and supply blood to the major organs, which apart from the brain continue to function normally. After a week or so, heart and circulation generally fail, following which vital organs are no longer viable for transplantation.

Increasingly, kidney transplant units are using kidneys from patients whose hearts have stopped and who have not been maintained on a ventilator (so called non-heart-beating donors). Once the circulation has stopped, the brain ceases to function after 3 minutes but the kidney remains viable and transplantable for up to 90 minutes.

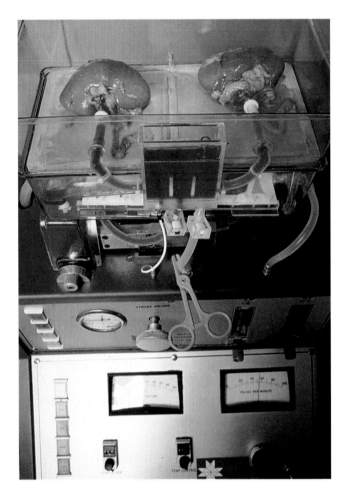

Donor kidneys
Two donor kidneys are preserved prior to transplantation. Both kidneys were taken from a cadaver donor. Each will be transplanted into a different recipient patient – the closest matches that can be found.

Living donors

The advantages of using a living related donor include:
• the possibility of an excellent or even a perfect match;
• the new kidney may be in a near-perfect condition;
• surgery for donor and recipient is planned in advance.
The outcome of transplantation from a living related well-matched donor is better than that from a cadaver donor. The risks to the donor have been estimated as 3 in 10,000 of the donor dying (0.03 per cent), and 1–2 in 100 of a significant surgical complication.

Laparoscopic kidney removal from a living donor

Four or five small incisions are made into the donor's abdomen. The surgeon inserts a video camera through one incision to view the kidney. Instruments needed to remove the kidney are inserted through two or three other openings. The kidney is cut free from its attachments, and severed tubes and vessels are clipped, stapled or tied. The kidney is scooped into a bag and extracted through another, larger, incision approximately 8cm (3in) long.

In contrast, open surgery to remove a kidney involves making a much larger incision in the patient's side and abdomen and spreading two ribs apart to remove the kidney. The discomfort suffered by the patient and the recovery time after surgery are both much greater than with laparoscopic surgery. But the success of any laparoscopic operation – and particularly such an advanced one as this – is dependent on the skill and experience of the surgeon in these new techniques.

In hospitals where surgeons are skilled and practised in the new laparoscopic techniques, laparoscopic kidney removal is by far the most popular option. In other hospitals, the safer and preferred option is still traditional open surgery.

❝

DONATING A KIDNEY

When my sister's kidneys had deteriorated to the extent that she required dialysis, our parents and I volunteered for tests to see whether any of us would be a suitable kidney donor.

It was me who turned out to be a positive match, since I had the same blood group as my sister and a sufficient number of matching antigens. A succession of tests followed, and once it was clear that there was no reason why my long-term health should suffer from the loss of a kidney, the date for the operation was set. The surgeon told me that she would be using the latest laparoscopic techniques, which would involve less discomfort and a quicker recovery time than with traditional open surgery.

I was admitted into hospital on the morning of the operation. I was in the operating theatre for four hours. When I woke up there were four incisions in my abdomen, the biggest being about 8cm (3in) long. I left the hospital three days later and was able to return to work three weeks after that. My sister is now fine, which made it all worth it.

❞

Transplanting a kidney

*A kidney transplantation involves two operating teams:
one team removes a kidney from the donor (dead or living),
then another team transplants the donated kidney into the
abdomen of the recipient.*

A kidney from a live donor is generally transplanted into the recipient's
abdomen within an hour of its removal from the donor. A kidney from a
donor who has died can be maintained in optimum condition for up to
48 hours. This is long enough for the kidney to be matched with the most
suitable recipient and then transported to the recipient's hospital.

The transplant operation usually takes about three hours. If there are no
complications or rejection episodes, the recipient might expect to spend a
week in hospital, followed by at least six weeks convalescence before
returning to work.

Success rates for kidney transplants

There is an 85–95 per cent chance that the kidney will still be working well
after a year. Thereafter new kidney grafts do fail at a rate of about 4 per cent
per year so that at five years and ten years the graft success rate is
approximately 70 per cent and 50 per cent respectively. Despite these overall
figures there are some well-matched kidneys (particularly those from close
blood relatives) that never experience any rejection episodes and are
functioning well for periods in excess of 20 years.

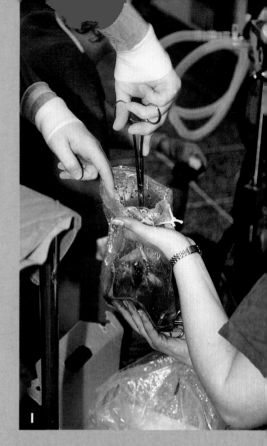

The surgical procedure

1 The donor kidney is unpacked. Since
its removal from the donor, it has been
kept inside a plastic bag, placed inside a
second bag, all within an insulated
polystyrene box containing crushed ice.

From two to three

Unless the failed kidneys pose a health
threat, they are left in place; the new
kidney is added to the two the recipient
already has – so the recipient ends up
with three kidneys. The new donor
kidney is generally positioned in the
lower abdomen, in the hollow of the
pelvis, on one side or the other. A renal
artery and vein from the donor kidney
are joined to the external iliac artery
and vein in the lower abdomen.

A section of ureter is also taken from
the donor along with the kidney, and this
is plumbed into the recipient's bladder
to take urine from the new kidney to
the bladder.

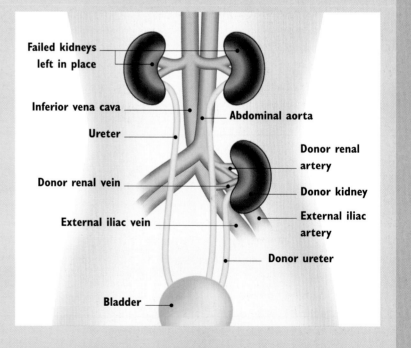

Failed kidneys
left in place

Inferior vena cava

Ureter

Donor renal vein

External iliac vein

Bladder

Abdominal aorta

Donor renal
artery

Donor kidney

External iliac
artery

Donor ureter

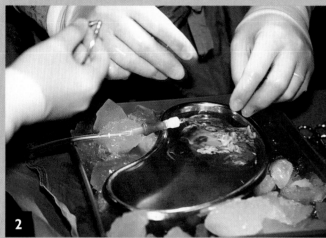

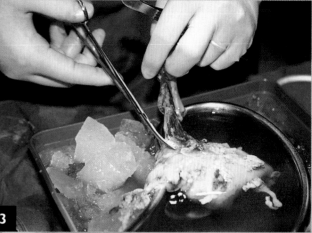

2 The kidney – in this case from a cadaver donor – must now be made ready for transplantation into the recipient. First it is flushed with perfusion solution, supplied through the tube at centre left. This is done to prepare the blood vessels for surgery

3 Then the excess fat is cut away. The kidney is still surrounded by ice to maintain its condition.

4 Having made an incision about 18cm (7in) long, and positioned the donor kidney in the patient's lower abdomen, the surgeon begins the delicate process of connecting the kidney's blood vessels to those of the patient. He works with clamps in place to stop bleeding from cut blood vessels.

5 The renal vein that belongs to the donor kidney is connected to an iliac vein, and the donor renal artery is attached to an iliac artery. Next, the clamps are released – if all is well, the kidney will suffuse with blood and turn pink. The donor ureter is then implanted in the bladder wall, so that urine from the new kidney will drain into the recipient's bladder. Once the surgeon is satisfied that the kidney is properly hooked up and functioning, he closes the incision.

6 A Doppler ultrasound scan checks venous (blue) and arterial (red) blood flow in the recently transplanted kidney. The kidney is the dark oval that fills most of the image.

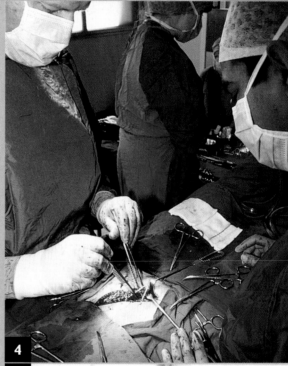

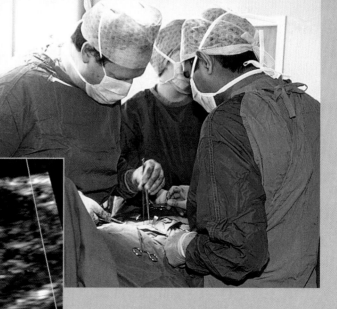

THE PROBLEM OF REJECTION

Following transplantation the donated kidney will be seen by the recipient's immune system as foreign and an attempt will be made to destroy the graft. The only exception is when a kidney is transplanted between identical twins. This rejection process has to be minimised by good tissue matching and suppressed by drugs.

IMMUNOSUPPRESSIVE DRUGS

The need for the patient to take immunosuppressive drugs throughout the life of the new kidney is the biggest source of complications following a transplant. This is because immunosuppressive drugs developed to prevent the rejection process also suppress and retard the beneficial aspects of the immune response. People who receive an organ transplant are therefore at risk of infections (often from organisms that do not normally attack healthy individuals) and a variety of virus-related cancers.

Which drugs are used?

Until the introduction of Cyclosporin A in the early 1980s steroids and Azathioprine were the only effective drugs available to prevent rejection. Such was the success of Cyclosporin A that by the late 1980s graft success rates

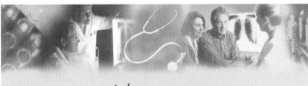

Milestones
IN MEDICINE

The first successful kidney transplant was carried out in Boston, USA, in 1954, when Ronald Herrick donated a kidney to his identical twin, Richard. Until that time, when the only alternative to a transplant was death, transplants had seemed promising but all recipients had died not long after surgery. Work in the early 1950s by British immunologist Peter Medawar on tissue rejection, and the Herricks' transplant in 1954, pointed the way forward. If a way to prevent the immune system rejecting foreign tissue could be found, a transplant might succeed in other cases too. At the end of the 1950s it was found that certain drugs could suppress the immune system, and a successful transplant between unrelated donors could be made.

had improved from 50 to 80 per cent at one year without any increase in complications. Since then, other effective immunosuppressive drugs have also been introduced.

- **Cyclosporin A** Cyclosporin A has been the backbone of immunosuppression for the last 20 years. However, side effects include diabetes, hypertension, raised cholesterol and an overgrowth of body hair and gums. In addition, the drug can damage kidneys, producing slow progressive scarring and ultimately can cause kidney failure. Careful measurement of blood levels and dose adjustments can minimise many of these side effects.
- **Tacrolimus** Developed in the late 1980s, Tacrolimus appears to be more powerful than Cyclosporin A. It does not produce overgrowth of hair and gums, but is more likely to cause diabetes.
- **Mycophenolate Mofetil** Since 1995 the addition of Mycophenolate Mofetil to both Cyclosporin A and Tacrolimus-based regimes reduced the incidence of acute rejection by about 20 per cent.
- **Sirolimus** This drug, the latest to be introduced, combines well with Tacrolimus, Cyclosporin A or Mycophenolate Mofetil. It seems to have the added benefit of reducing fibrosis and scarring and so may be of great value in preventing poorly functioning grafts from experiencing chronic rejection.

Typically, patients are given Cyclosporin A or Tacrolimus combined with Azathioprine or Mycophenolate, plus steroids, but doctors always tailor immunosuppressive regimes to the needs of the individual patient. Sirolimus or Mycophenolate can be added to counter chronic rejection. Fewer and fewer steroids are being used as newer, more potent drugs are developed.

Antibody therapy

Antibodies to the cells of the human immune system can be given to a patient intravenously immediately after the transplant operation. These agents are powerful and have an important role in preventing rejection, particularly in patients who have had a previous transplant, and also in reversing very aggressive rejection crises.

AFTER A KIDNEY TRANSPLANT

All kidney transplant patients need life-long medical follow-up and careful supervision of their complex drug regimes, but when a graft is stable and functions well there may be no more than two or three outpatient visits a year to the hospital.

Cloning for 'spare' organs

The biggest limitation on the number of transplant operations is the limited number of suitable donor organs. This is true not just for kidney transplants, but for all organ transplant programmes. As more of us live into old age, so the chances of one of our organs failing increases, and the demand for transplant surgery goes up. To overcome this shortfall in available donor organs, various genetic techniques are being researched. If successful, these could revolutionise transplant surgery.

One such technique is cloning. This involves making a genetically identical copy of a single cell, or organ, or even a whole individual. There has been a great deal of debate on this subject since the birth in Scotland in 1996 of Dolly, the first cloned sheep (above). It may in the future be possible to clone and grow a healthy organ from a person's own cells, if they were to be removed from their body and grown in a laboratory. These could then be transplanted back into the body in exchange for a diseased, failing organ, with the huge advantage that the patient's own immune system would not try to reject the organ, as it would recognise it as its own. This would avoid the need for the powerful anti-rejection drugs, which have to be taken at present to suppress the immune system.

Another line of research that seeks to produce a limitless supply of organs for transplantation, without the organs provoking a rejection response, is by using so-called transgenic animals. The research involves altering the animals' genes by 'splicing in' new human genetic information. The theory is that the human body will not detect organs 'donated' by transgenic animals as being 'foreign'. Research into how to produce transgenic pigs for use as organ donors for humans is already well underway in the UK and USA. This area of research is full of ethical dilemmas, however, and discussion on these issues is likely to continue for years to come.

A successful, stable kidney transplant restores good health and vitality to a patient. Diet and fluid allowances can be relaxed. Anaemia and bone disease recover. In women menstrual cycles return and pregnancy becomes possible. There is usually an improvement in heart function.

When the new kidney functions poorly or fails

Some patients do experience a moderate degree of kidney failure after a transplant. Such patients need treatment to control the complications of kidney impairment and to stop rejection of their transplant. A graft that functions poorly at six months after transplant may only last a year or two. If a graft ultimately fails, most patients are usually fit and well enough to return to dialysis and eventually – hopefully – receive a new transplant.

Continuing medical problems

About half of all patients who have undergone a kidney transplant continue to experience medical problems associated with the diseases that caused kidney failure in the first place. This is especially the case with patients who have developed the complications associated with diabetes; a kidney transplant in itself does not improve the non-kidney complications of diabetes.

The long-term side effects of immunosuppression

Some patients will suffer from the side effects of immunosuppressive drugs: notably high blood pressure, diabetes and/or raised blood cholesterol. These side effects can lead to accelerating circulatory diseases (strokes, heart attacks and heart failure). Indeed, the most common causes of death following transplantation are diseases of the heart and circulation. This is also true for patients on long-term dialysis. As a result, many patients will need to take a regime of drugs to reduce the risks of heart and circulatory diseases, as well as immunosuppressive drugs to prevent rejection of the kidney.

Transplant patients also run the risk of skin cancers, and as a result special dermatology clinics dedicated to their needs have been established.

Removing a diseased or damaged kidney

Performing a nephrectomy – the surgical removal of an entire kidney – is never undertaken lightly. The usual causes are a cancerous growth in the kidney or the kidney having become damaged beyond repair as a result of injury – from a stabbing, perhaps, or a gunshot wound.

BEFORE THE OPERATION

Cancer may be suspected if a solid mass is detected in one or other kidney on an ultrasound scan or intravenous urogram (IVU). More precise information about the exact site and size of the mass would then be gained by performing a computed tomogram (CT) scan. This would also give much needed information on any possible spread of the cancer to nearby organs. This information is essential to the surgeons planning such an operation so that they will know what to expect once in the operating theatre and inside the body.

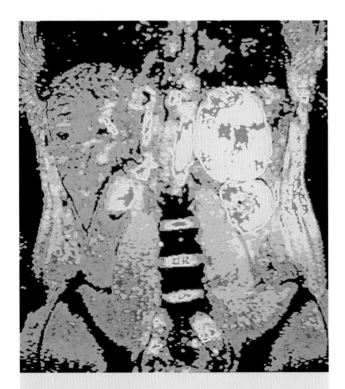

Cancer of the kidney

Coloured magnetic resonance imaging (MRI) reveals a vertical slice through the abdomen of a sufferer from cancer of the kidney. A large cancerous tumour is clearly visible above one of the kidneys. Both kidneys and tumour are shown in yellow. Between the kidneys lie vertebrae belonging to the spinal cord.

How does one kidney cope with the work of two?

A patient facing the removal of a kidney is naturally concerned to know how their body will cope with only the one kidney. In fact, the body copes surprisingly well. The other kidney enlarges slightly and has enough functional reserve to be able to take over most of the work of the lost organ, so that there is little, if any, noticeable change as far as the patient is concerned.

ASK THE EXPERT

THE OPERATION

A variety of different incisions are used to gain access to the kidneys, including a cut in the flank, just below the ribs, and a cut straight up and down the abdomen in the middle, from beneath the centre of the rib cage down to below the navel.

A cancer-free ureter is tied off but left in place. If cancer involves a ureter as well as a kidney, then the ureter has to be traced right down to the bladder and removed. All blood vessels going to and from the kidney are tied off and cut so that the kidney can be removed. Generally a radical nephrectomy is performed if there is cancer, in which case the associated adrenal gland and the fat surrounding the kidney are also removed.

When cancer has spread beyond the kidney

Lymph nodes close to the kidney are removed, because the lymphatic system is one of the commonest routes by which all cancers spread around the body. One unusual feature of kidney cancer is that it can spread by growing up the veins. These blood vessels must be explored for signs of tumour spread and removed as necessary.

If surgery reveals that the cancer has spread beyond the kidney, then external beam radiotherapy may be used as a supplementary treatment once the patient has recovered from the immediate after-effects of the operation.

Major bladder surgery

Surgeons only resort to major surgery on the bladder as a treatment for urinary incontinence if all other alternatives have been tried and found wanting. This is because of the risk – sometimes a certainty – of unwanted side effects.

CLAM CYSTOPLASTY

Clam cystoplasty is an operation in which the bladder is cut open, then augmented with a section from the small intestine that has been opened out before being sewn into place. The purpose is to improve bladder overactivity by 'damping down' unstable waves of contraction in the bladder. This means that the pressure doesn't rise to the point where the patient is unable to prevent urine from leaving the bladder.

During the operation there is a risk of bowel obstruction and bleeding. Later, there may be difficulties emptying the bladder, or recurrent urinary tract infections. For these reasons this operation is an option only if all alternatives – bladder training, behavioural therapy and anticholinergic drugs – have been explored first without success. But some patients with very overactive bladders do find that this operation provides overall benefit.

CYSTECTOMY AND URINARY DIVERSION

Occasionally, operations are performed to divert the passage of urine flow away from its normal path from kidneys to bladder to urethra. They are needed following the removal of the bladder (a cystectomy) as a treatment for bladder cancer. They are very occasionally employed as treatments for urinary incontinence, but only after all other treatments have been found to be inadequate.

A bladder is generally removed entirely; sometimes, if a cancerous tumour is confined to one region of the bladder, it is only partially removed. A total, or radical, cystectomy involves first cutting and tying the ureters that attach the bladder to the kidneys, then removing associated organs as well as the bladder itself. In women the uterus, fallopian tubes, ovaries and cervix are removed too; in men, the prostate gland is cut out.

With urinary diversion, there are several options.
- **Surface diversion** The two ureters are connected to a newly created 'bladder' formed from a section of small intestine. Alternatively, a continent diversion is created, in which urine is stored in the new bladder and drained out via a catheter inserted through an outlet in the skin.
- **Diverting urine into the bowel** Urine is diverted so that it drains into the large intestine and is expelled from the body along with the faeces. This can lead to infections that may spread to the kidneys and so is not often used.

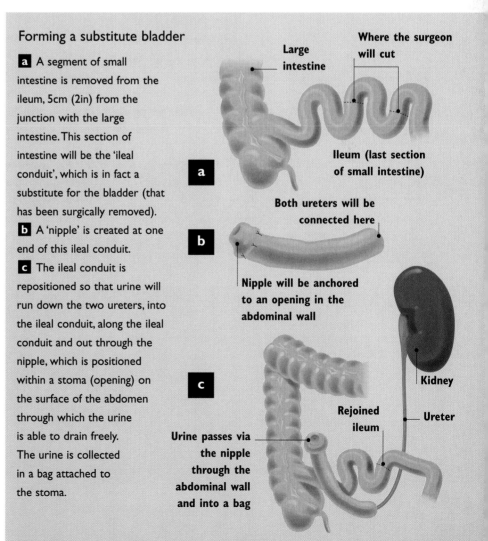

Forming a substitute bladder

a A segment of small intestine is removed from the ileum, 5cm (2in) from the junction with the large intestine. This section of intestine will be the 'ileal conduit', which is in fact a substitute for the bladder (that has been surgically removed).

b A 'nipple' is created at one end of this ileal conduit.

c The ileal conduit is repositioned so that urine will run down the two ureters, into the ileal conduit, along the ileal conduit and out through the nipple, which is positioned within a stoma (opening) on the surface of the abdomen through which the urine is able to drain freely. The urine is collected in a bag attached to the stoma.

Large intestine

Where the surgeon will cut

Ileum (last section of small intestine)

Both ureters will be connected here

Nipple will be anchored to an opening in the abdominal wall

Kidney

Rejoined ileum

Ureter

Urine passes via the nipple through the abdominal wall and into a bag

Prostate operations

The purpose of operating on a man's prostate gland is generally to relieve uncomfortable symptoms arising from an enlarged prostate. This condition is usually benign, but it can be due to prostate cancer, in which case the operation will attempt to remove the cancer as well.

The prostate gland is a male accessory sex gland positioned at the base of the bladder. During ejaculation it secretes into the urethra an alkaline fluid that is a key constituent of semen. The fact that it surrounds the urethra means that if the prostate enlarges, the urethra becomes squeezed. This obstructs the flow of urine from the bladder, which then has to contract with more force than before in order to empty. The effect of this is to cause the bladder muscle wall to thicken. The increased pressure can also cause damage to the urinary tract higher up.

Symptoms arising from a partially obstructed urethra include poor urinary flow, a frequent and insistent urge to urinate, and dribbling from the penis end after passing urine.

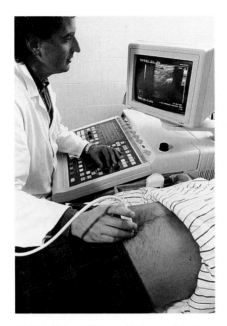

Viewing the prostate gland
A doctor uses ultrasound scanning to examine a patient's prostate gland. The transducer held against the patient's abdomen emits sound waves that echo off internal structures.

TRANSURETHRAL RESECTION OF THE PROSTATE (TURP)

This common urological operation is a laparoscopic procedure that involves passing an operating cystoscope (often called a resectoscope) up the urethra from the tip of the penis while the patient is under a general anaesthetic. The surgeon uses the resectoscope to cut pieces from the enlarged prostate in order to clear a channel for urine to drain freely from the bladder.

Before the operation

The decision on whether to perform this operation is dependent on the extent of obstruction at the bladder neck caused by the enlarged prostate gland, and whether there is any evidence that any part of the upper urinary tract is being damaged as a result of pressure from urine backing up the ureters. If obstruction is not severe and cancer not suspected, then drug treatment can be used instead, to try to slow down or reverse the growth of the prostate.

Investigations can be made prior to surgery to try to determine whether the enlarged prostate gland is benign or malignant. These include a rectal examination, measuring 'tumour markers' in the blood, and a trans-rectal ultrasound scan of the prostate. However, it is not until the operation is over that the exact cause can be identified; the transurethral resection itself provides the sample that is sent off for a biopsy.

The effect of an enlarged prostate

a The prostate gland is positioned immediately below the bladder, with the urethra running through its centre. When normal size, it does not impede the flow of urine in any way.

b As men age, the prostate gland slowly enlarges. This leads to the urethra becoming squeezed and – eventually – partially blocked.

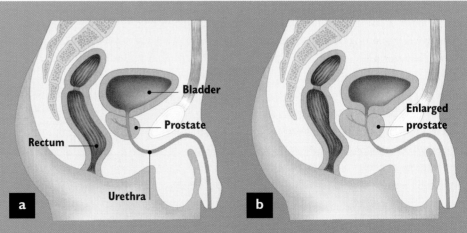

Bladder

Prostate

Rectum

Urethra

a

Enlarged prostate

b

During the operation

A system of lenses and fibreoptics provides a high-definition video image of the view through the resectoscope. The surgeon can see this on a video monitor in the operating theatre. Sterile fluid is circulated down the resectoscope, around the bladder and urethra and back up the instrument by means of a pump. This keeps the field of vision clear and carries away any debris.

Firstly the bladder is inspected for signs of thickening of the muscle wall. Then the bladder neck and the section of the urethra that runs through the prostate are assessed. The resectoscope has a loop of wire that can be heated by an electric current to act as a small cutting tool. This is used to 'chip away' at the enlarged prostate. The 'chippings' are sent to a pathologist to be analysed for any signs of cancer.

In recent years alternatives to resecting the prostate with a loop of hot wire have emerged. These include the use of lasers and microwave energy at the tip of the cystoscope to clear a channel within the urethra.

After the operation

Postoperative bleeding from the prostate can be a problem in the first few days after surgery. For this reason a catheter is left in the bladder for several days whilst sterile fluid is used to irrigate the operative site. This prevents the build-up of blood clots, which would block off the bladder neck.

Other longer-term risks of transurethral resection include impotence (in about one in six of all cases), urinary incontinence (about 1 per cent of cases) and retrograde ejaculation. This latter means that semen no longer ejaculates from the penis tip, but enters the bladder instead. It is common following this procedure, though not dangerous. For these reasons it is better that a patient has completed his family before having this operation.

Despite these relative risks, this operation greatly improves the quality of life of most patients. Sometimes the prostate grows again and the operation has to be repeated after a few years, if symptoms cannot be controlled by drug treatment alone.

PROSTATECTOMY

This is the removal of the entire male prostate gland. It may be recommended if the prostate is so large that a transurethral resection is not practical, or if cancer of the prostate is suspected and 'aggressive' treatment to remove

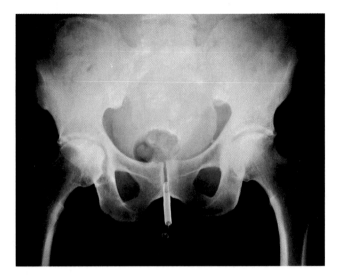

Prostatic implant
The implant shown on this coloured X-ray has been inserted high up in the urethra, in the region of the prostate gland. This device is used to relieve bladder obstruction caused by an enlarged prostate.

the entire gland plus the regional lymph nodes is thought to offer the best chance of a cure. These lymph nodes are removed too because the lymphatic system is one of the commonest routes by which all cancers spread around the body. This operation is known as a radical prostatectomy and is increasingly used if the prostate cancer has not spread too far by the time it is diagnosed.

As when planning any surgery, it is extremely important to get as much information as possible before operating. This is obtained by measuring 'tumour markers' in the blood, noting the texture and size of the prostate on rectal examination and by the use of imaging techniques.

The operation can be performed using laparoscopic methods or open surgery. The entire prostate gland is removed, and then sent to a pathologist for further examination. A catheter is usually left in the bladder for several days to allow the bladder time to rest, and the patient should expect to be in hospital for up to a week after the operation.

The prostate gland is very well supplied with blood vessels and because of this, blood loss during the operation can be considerable. This may result in the patient requiring a blood transfusion. Possible damage to the bladder neck and sphincter muscle, which are important in maintaining continence, is also a risk. Approximately one in twelve men become incontinent after a total prostatectomy. It is likely that there will be at least some loss of sexual function as well.

Other cancer treatments

The first line of treatment for cancers of the kidneys, bladder and urinary tract is, if at all possible, surgery. Other procedures – performed either alone or before or after surgery – include radiotherapy, chemotherapy and, in cases of prostate cancer, hormone treatment.

Planning the most suitable method of treating any case of cancer involves careful calculation and a high degree of skill and experience on behalf of the medical and surgical experts involved (see page 97). Surgical intervention often has to be supported by other forms of treatment. Radiotherapy and chemotherapy are often crucial pre and post-operative treatments where cancer is the problem. In addition, drug therapy often goes hand in hand with surgery, as with the use of drugs to regulate testosterone production in prostate cancer patients, for example.

CANCER WITHIN THE KIDNEY

Renal cell cancer arising in the kidneys – the causes of which are largely unknown – is usually treated by surgical removal of the tumour, which may well involve removing the entire kidney. Radiotherapy may be administered after the operation if the cancer was not completely removed. There is no effective chemotherapy treatment.

Hot and cold probes

Some surgeons are now using probes inserted through the skin to kill cancer cells by burning or freezing cells until they are dead. In the procedure called percutaneous radiofrequency ablation (PRA), a radiofrequency generator very precisely heats the tip of the probe so that it can kill cancer cells while harming as little surrounding tissue as possible. This technique has proved particularly useful on kidney and liver tumours. A cryoprobe employs cold rather than heat to kill prostate cancer cells.

The ice ball at the tip of the cryoprobe shown here (next to its control panel) cools in seconds to -90°C (-130°F) to destroy cancer cells by freezing them.

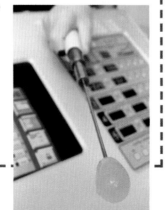

BLADDER CANCER

Superficial tumours may be cut or burned away; less commonly, they are treated by chemotherapy alone. Invasive tumours that have penetrated more deeply into the bladder wall and maybe spread beyond to the lymph nodes or even further are often treated by removing the bladder entirely (see page 129), with radiotherapy or chemotherapy as follow-up treatments if necessary.

TUMOURS IN THE URETHRA

Tumours in the urethra occur much less often than bladder cancer; they can be caused by the spread of cancer from the bladder, or follow on from chronic inflammation. They may be treated with radiotherapy alone, with the aim of clearing the tract of tumours.

CANCER OF THE PROSTATE

Cancerous tumours within the prostate gland in men are treated with transurethral resection of the prostate (see page 130) if caught early. Advanced tumours may require a prostatectomy and/or radiotherapy.

More than three-quarters of prostate cancers are found to need the hormone testosterone to grow. If the cancer has spread beyond the prostate gland, hormone treatment may be used to arrest the cancer's spread: the production of testosterone can be suppressed by drugs or depleted by surgery (by removing the testicles).

If hormone treatment eventually proves ineffective, chemotherapy may be the next step. 'Palliative' radiotherapy is sometimes used to treat bone pain, caused by the spread of 'secondary' cancers to the bones from a 'primary' prostate (or kidney) cancer.

An alternative treatment for a cancer growth that has not spread beyond the prostate is brachytherapy, in which tiny pellets of radioactive metal or iodine are implanted within the prostate gland. The implant is made by inserting a long needle through the abdomen wall, or through the perineum behind the base of the penis. The pellets are able to deliver a higher dose of radiation to the tumour than would be the case with conventional external beam radiation therapy.

A TO Z

OF DISEASES AND DISORDERS

This section gives information on the main illnesses and medical conditions that can affect the kidneys and urinary system.

This index is arranged alphabetically and each entry is structured in a similar way:

What are the causes?

What are the symptoms?

How is it diagnosed?

What are the treatment options?

How can it be prevented or minimised?

What is the outlook?

ACUTE NEPHRITIC SYNDROME

The abrupt development of oedema (swelling, particularly around the ankles), protein in the urine (proteinuria), red blood cells in the urine (haematuria), high blood pressure and impaired kidney function.

What are the causes?

There are many causes of acute nephritic syndrome, including infection, and the treatment and prognosis cannot be stated with confidence unless a more definitive diagnosis is established. The association between this syndrome and infection of the skin or pharynx with streptococci bacteria has been known for a century. Acute nephritic syndrome of this type is known as post-infectious glomerulonephritis and although this condition is now uncommon in developed countries it remains a substantial problem in the developing nations.

How is it diagnosed?

Red cells present in the urine because of inflammation in the kidney have an abnormal appearance, which becomes evident when a sample of urine is examined under a microscope. Because so many conditions can contribute to the syndrome, it is often necessary to undertake a kidney biopsy to make a precise diagnosis.

What are the treatment options?

Treatment may involve bed rest, antibiotics and limiting salt in the diet. Corticosteroids, or other anti-inflammatory drugs, may be prescribed.

What is the outlook?

Most cases of post-infectious glomerulonephritis have a good outcome with eventual recovery of renal function.

ACUTE PYELONEPHRITIS

A sudden and severe infection within the kidney.

What are the causes?

Infection reaches the kidney by ascending from the opening of the urethra into the bladder and then up the ureter into the kidney itself. Acute pyelonephritis usually follows, or is associated with, infection of the bladder (cystitis). In some patients there is an anatomical abnormality that predisposes to infection, such as a kidney stone, congenital abnormalities, reflux (backflow of urine from the bladder) or impaired bladder emptying.

What are the symptoms?

Patients feel unwell and feverish and sometimes develop attacks of shivering. There is usually pain and tenderness over the affected kidney. If the infection is unchecked, blood pressure may fall and septic shock can develop if the infection spreads to the bloodstream.

What are the treatment options?

Treatment is with high-dose intravenous antibiotics, given in hospital. It may be necessary to give intravenous fluids for a few days to correct or prevent dehydration. Antibiotics will usually be continued by mouth for at least four weeks, or two weeks after any tenderness of the kidney has resolved, whichever is the longer. Once the acute episode has passed a full urological evaluation should be undertaken to check any predisposing causes that may require treatment.

ACUTE RENAL FAILURE

See Kidney failure, p. 145.

ALPORT'S SYNDROME

A genetically inherited condition experienced by some families involving haematuria (blood in the urine), deafness and progressive renal failure.

In 1927, Dr Cecil Alport described successive generations of a family with symptoms of haematuria, deafness and renal failure. By recording the family history he noticed a difference in the extent to which the disease affected the sexes: 'males develop nephritis and deafness and do not as a rule survive', whereas 'females have deafness and haematuria, and live to old age'. This pattern, characteristic of X-linked dominant inheritance is still found in 85–90 per cent of the families who have Alport's syndrome.

What are the causes?

Defects in part of the glomerular basement membrane (GBM) called type IV collagen have been identified, as have the genes that code for type IV collagen. Defects most commonly occur in a gene on the X chromosome, one of the chromosomes which determine a person's sex, and this explains the pattern of inheritance that Alport described. Less commonly the defect can occur in genes on a non-sex determining chromosome. Different defects or mutations occur in different families and this may be reflected in the severity of the symptoms.

What are the symptoms?

High-frequency hearing loss is usually present. Problems with the lens and retina of the eye can occur in up to 40 per cent of individuals, but these do not usually compromise vision. The main feature in the kidney is blood in the urine. Protein in the urine may also be found in some patients and may be heavy enough to cause nephrotic syndrome (p. 147). In adults, high blood pressure or abnormalities in kidney function are often the first signs to be spotted.

How is it diagnosed?

Hearing defects may be mild and in some cases only detected after special testing. Blood may be apparent only when the urine is examined under the microscope or tested with dipsticks. Visible blood may occur in children, but is unusual in adults. Blood tests can check for high blood pressure or abnormalities in kidney function.

What are the treatment options?

Hearing loss can be improved with a hearing aid. When the disease has progressed to the extent that a patient has chronic renal failure, dialysis and kidney transplantation provide highly effective life-sustaining treatment.

What is the outlook?

The rate at which kidney function deteriorates varies. It is unusual for dialysis to be required before the age of 10 years old, and although many affected individuals begin dialysis in their 40s, it may not be required until much later. Female Alport's carriers are relatively mildly affected, although 5–15 per cent may require dialysis. Alport's early description of the syndrome suggested that males do not usually survive, but the introduction of dialysis and kidney transplantation now means that the outlook is good.

BEDWETTING

See Nocturnal enuresis, p. 148.

BENIGN PROSTATIC HYPERTROPHY

A common condition, benign prostatic hypertrophy (BPH) causes the prostate gland in men slowly to increase in size, over a number of years.

Enlargement of the prostate gland seems to be an inevitable consequence of getting older. By the age of 50, almost 50 per cent of men are affected by BPH, and by the age of 80 this figure has risen to more than 90 per cent. This is not a worry in itself, since the growth is not malignant and will not spread around the body, in the way that a cancer does.

What are the causes?

The exact cause is unknown. A popular theory is that this increase in size is due to changing hormone levels in men as they get older, especially the increasing accumulation in the prostate of the male hormone dihydrotestosterone.

What are the symptoms?

Although the prostate starts to enlarge by the age of 40, it is a slow process and symptoms do not commonly appear until the ages of 50 to 70, when the enlarged prostate starts to obstruct the male urethra. The commonest, and usually the first, symptom to appear is increased frequency in passing urine. This is accompanied by other 'irritative' bladder symptoms of urinary urgency and nocturia (needing to get up frequently in the night to pass urine). Initially the bladder compensates for the obstruction by contracting more powerfully, but as the prostate continues to enlarge, eventually the rate of flow is affected. This leads to difficulty in starting to pass urine and a poor stream that dribbles to nothing as it finishes. If the outflow from the bladder becomes blocked, this leads to acute urinary retention. BHP has a detrimental effect on a number of measures of the quality of life, including sleeping patterns, mobility, sexual function and sense of well-being.

How is it diagnosed?

Benign prostatic hypertrophy should always be considered likely in any man over the age of 50 with these symptoms. The other major disease that causes the prostate to enlarge, and hence causes similar symptoms, is prostate cancer, which is much less common. In making a diagnosis it is important to tell the conditions apart. A rectal examination allows the back of the prostate gland to be felt: in BPH the gland feels enlarged, firm and rubbery. Blood tests are taken to look for the presence of prostate specific antigen (PSA), a 'tumour marker' that is usually raised in prostate cancer. If diagnosis is uncertain, a biopsy may be taken and a transrectal ultrasound scan performed. It is also important to investigate the effect these may have on the upper urinary tract (kidneys and ureters). This is done through blood tests to check renal function and an intravenous urogram (p. 102) or ultrasound scan to image the upper tract. A midstream urine sample will also be tested to ensure that the obstruction has not caused a urinary tract infection.

What are the treatment options?

How best to treat the condition depends on the severity of the symptoms, the age and general health of the patient, and whether damage is being done to the upper urinary tract as a result of obstruction. There are various options.

• No immediate treatment, but monitor the patient's condition and state of health carefully.

• Different types of drug therapy, such as alpha blockers that relax the muscle tone in the bladder neck and so help to relieve the obstruction. Finasteride, which prevents the formation of the hormone dihydrotestosterone, shrinks the size of the prostate when taken for more than six months.

• Surgery to carry out either a transurethral resection of the prostate (TURP) or, if the prostate is particularly enlarged, a prostatectomy (removal of the prostate gland).

What is the outlook?

Nothing clearly reduces the likelihood of developing BPH. However, the potentially damaging effects on the upper urinary tract if the condition goes unchecked can be prevented. After diagnosis, the function of the kidneys can be monitored and symptoms greatly reduced. Surgery can affect sexual function, although experts disagree on how many men are affected, and the extent to which they have problems. Most men who were able to sustain an erection before surgery can do so afterwards, although surgery is unable to restore function to those who have lost it already. Surgery usually causes retrograde ejaculation (p. 153).

BLADDER TUMOURS

Bladder tumours, like all tumours of the urinary tract, are more common in men than in women.

Some 98 per cent of bladder tumours are malignant, but many are slow growing and do not spread aggressively. Around 12,000 new cases of bladder cancer are diagnosed in England and Wales each year, making it the second most common urological cancer, after prostate cancer.

What are the causes?

Historically, there is a very strong link between bladder cancer and a particular group of chemicals found in the dye and rubber industries. Health and safety regulations make this less of a risk today. Bladder cancer is linked to cigarette smoking – it is estimated that smoking increases the risk of developing bladder cancer as much as four times. By far the biggest risk factor worldwide is infection with the parasitic worm schistosomiasis, which is commonly found in much of the developing world. This causes the disease bilharzia and greatly increases the risk of developing a particular type of bladder cancer known as squamous cell carcinoma.

What are the symptoms?

In the initial stages there may not be any symptoms. The classic symptom associated with bladder tumours is the passage of blood in the urine (haematuria). This is usually painless but always calls for further investigation, both of the bladder and the upper urinary tract. Visible haematuria is a feature of 90 per cent of bladder cancers. In a further 5–10 per cent of cases smaller amounts of blood are present in the urine, but not apparent to the naked eye. Both types of haematuria may be intermittent in cases of bladder cancer. This means that even if blood in the urine appears to 'clear up' there may still be an underlying cause, which needs prompt investigation.

If a lot of blood flows into the bladder, this may lead to pain and difficulty passing urine, since blood clots can block urine flow. Generally, however, pain is a late symptom.

How is it diagnosed?

Bladder tumours are suspected from the symptoms. The diagnosis is confirmed by a cystoscopy to look inside the bladder (p. 106). Any suspicious-looking growths can be removed and sent to a pathologist for a definitive diagnosis. The upper urinary tracts are assessed with an ultrasound or an IVU, since cancer of the ureters or the kidneys can cause similar symptoms. A CT or MRI scan may be useful if it is felt that the cancer may have spread beyond the bladder.

What are the treatment options?

Treatment depends on the type of tumour and how advanced it is. If the tumour is benign or an early-stage malignant tumour, removing it during the cystoscopy is often sufficient. More advanced stages require more radical treatment. This can take the form of a surgical cystectomy (removing the bladder and diverting the flow of urine), external beam radiotherapy or chemotherapy. If treatment fails to eradicate the cancer, or the extent of the disease at diagnosis is such that a cure is not possible, palliative treatment can make a patient more comfortable and prolong survival, without the expectation of a cure.

How can it be prevented or minimised?

The chances of developing a bladder tumour can be reduced by not smoking. By seeking early advice and further investigation for blood in the urine, it is more likely that if bladder cancer is present, it will be picked up early. This gives the best hope of a successful outcome to treatment.

BRIGHT'S DISEASE
See *Acute nephritic syndrome, p. 134;*
Glomerulonephritis, p. 139.

CHRONIC PYELONEPHRITIS
See *Reflux nephropathy, p. 152.*

CHRONIC RENAL FAILURE
See *Kidney failure, p. 145.*

CONGENITAL NEPHROTIC SYNDROME
A rare inherited disorder characterised by protein in the urine and fluid retention.

What are the causes?
The syndrome mainly affects people of Finnish origin, and is inherited autosomal recessively, so that both parents must possess a defective copy of the responsible gene for a child to develop the condition. Proteinuria (protein in the urine) develops before birth or soon afterwards. This loss of protein into the urine includes antibodies against infection, resulting in frequent infections and malnutrition. Swelling around the eyes and of the stomach and legs is common.

What are the treatment options?
Management of affected children should be undertaken in a specialist paediatric nephrology centre. The prognosis for affected children is poor, although early kidney transplantation has proven successful for some children.

CYSTOCELE
A pelvic organ prolapse: the bladder bulges into the top of the vagina, giving the sensation of a lump in the vagina.

Cystocele is often found with other types of prolapse in the vagina, such as the uterus descending into the vagina (uterine prolapse) or the rectum bulging into the vagina (rectocele). The condition is common in post-menopausal women and is linked with symptoms such as stress incontinence.

What are the causes?
A cystocele is caused by a lack of support in holding the pelvic organs in their correct position. There is no one cause but a number of factors that make this more likely. These include being overweight, smoking and having experienced a difficult birth, particularly if the pushing stage of labour was long, or if the baby was large. Age is a risk factor, since the muscles and ligaments become weaker with age, especially after the menopause. There is a strong genetic element, which determines how strong the supporting tissues are, and hence the risk of developing a prolapse. Occasionally a cystocele results from the bladder being pushed down on to the vagina by a mass, such as a large cyst on an ovary.

What are the symptoms?
In milder forms there are usually no symptoms. As the bladder bulges further into the vagina, the woman becomes more aware of the feeling that there is a lump there, especially when bearing down or coughing. The sensation is frequently worse at the end of the day, or after standing for a long time. It may become more difficult to empty the bladder, and urine may leak out when coughing or sneezing as the neck of the bladder is pulled out of position.

How is it diagnosed?
A cystocele is diagnosed by vaginal examination. This may be done with the patient in both a lying and a standing position to get an idea of the severity of the cystocele and any other types of pelvic organ prolapse. A physical examination is also necessary to ensure that the prolapse is not the result of a large abdominal or pelvic mass, such as a cyst, pushing down on the bladder. If there is concern

Can HRT help prevent a cystocele?

Lack of oestrogen after the menopause can contribute to the formation of a cystocele, and many experts believe that hormone replacement therapy (HRT) can help to maintain the strength of the tissues that support the pelvic organs, including the bladder, in post-menopausal women. However, oestrogen cannot reverse a prolapse once it is already there. In addition, oestrogen replacement is not suitable for every woman, so doctors will tailor treatment to an individual case.

ASK THE EXPERT

that this may be the case, or if the examination is difficult because the patient is overweight, an ultrasound scan of the pelvis is performed. Any urinary symptoms such as stress incontinence are best investigated with urodynamic tests (p. 101). A midstream urine sample (MSU) should also be analysed to ensure that inefficient emptying of the bladder has not caused a urinary tract infection.

What are the treatment options?

Small cystoceles that are not causing any symptoms are usually left untreated, although pelvic floor physiotherapy may be of benefit in some cases. If the cystocele is large and the patient is aware of a lump, or has urinary symptoms connected with it, surgery offers the best treatment. Although a cystocele is not life threatening, it can severely interfere with quality of life and surgical correction offers very good cure rates. An alternative for someone who does not wish to have an operation, or who is too unwell to undergo surgery, is the use of a vaginal ring pessary. This device is fitted into the vagina to provide support for the bladder. It needs to be replaced every six months.

How can it be prevented or minimised?

The chance of getting a cystocele, or indeed any form of prolapse, can be minimised by attempting to reduce the known risk factors. Careful management of women in labour lessens the risk both of prolapse in later life and of bladder damage. Maintaining a sensible weight and level of physical activity reduces the risk, as does not smoking.

CYSTITIS
See Urinary tract infection, p. 154.

DETRUSOR SPHINCTER DYSSYNERGIA
A disorder caused by neurological damage to the finely coordinated system of nerves that supply the bladder.

Bladder function involves storing urine produced by the kidneys, and releasing it when convenient. When the bladder contracts, the nerves instruct the urethral sphincter muscle, which closes off the outflow from the bladder, to relax and so allow urine to be passed. If this coordination is lost and the urethral sphincter remains closed, the bladder has to generate enormous force to overcome the obstruction. The bladder becoming thicker and more muscular, and increases the likelihood of vesicoureteric reflux (p. 154).

What are the causes?

A variety of neurological conditions can cause DSD, including spina bifida, multiple sclerosis, spinal cord injuries and tumours pressing on the spinal cord.

What are the symptoms?

The dysfunction of the bladder neck causes difficulties with passing urine, and flow rate may be intermittent and reduced. Symptoms depend on the type of neurological condition responsible for DSD. Urinary incontinence is frequently a problem because the bladder starts to contract spontaneously. Other neurological symptoms are often present, such as muscle weakness, visual disturbance and difficulty in coordinating movements. The combination of bladder and neurological symptoms should be investigated.

How is it diagnosed?

In diagnosing DSD, it is important not only to assess the degree of bladder dysfunction, but also to look for the underlying neurological disease. This may be obvious in some patients because the neurological diagnosis may have already been made before the onset of bladder symptoms. Alternatively, the bladder symptoms may be the start of an undiagnosed neurological condition. DSD is diagnosed using urodynamic tests. Videocystometrography is useful as the urethral sphincter can be seen to contract on X-ray imaging at the same time as the bladder is shown to be contracting. Vesicoureteric reflux may be a consequence of DSD and can also be looked for during videocystometrography. A specialist neurologist is required to diagnose the wider neurological problem through neurological examination and imaging of the brain and spine.

What are the treatment options?

Choice of treatment depends on the underlying cause. If the cause can be treated – for instance, by removing a tumour – the bladder symptoms are likely to improve. But often this is not the case. Symptoms can be treated to improve quality of life and reduce the risk of damage to the upper urinary tract from obstruction and vesicoureteric reflux. This is achieved by enabling the bladder to drain more efficiently by clean intermittent self-catheterisation, insertion of a suprapubic catheter, or by neuromodulation (p. 112).

How can it be prevented or minimised?

Little can be done to prevent the causes of DSD, but it is important that this disorder is diagnosed and treated in order to prevent further damage higher up the urinary tract.

DIABETES

This disorder, also known as diabetes mellitus, is one of the most common causes of kidney failure in the developed world.

Diabetes affects the body's ability to regulate glucose, needed to produce energy. When diabetes occurs in childhood or adolescence, it is called type I. This results from the failure of the pancreas gland to produce the hormone insulin, usually because cells in the pancreas have been attacked by the body's own immune system. In later life, type II diabetes is more common. Here, the pancreas does produce insulin but the cells of the body do not respond normally to it. Both forms of diabetes cause complications in many parts of the body, including the eyes, nerves, blood vessels and kidneys.

What are the causes?

The exact mechanism through which diabetes damages kidneys is not known, but it is probably related to the prolonged effects of abnormally high glucose in the blood. The main damage occurs in the glomeruli. Diabetes can also cause atherosclerosis, a build-up of fatty deposits in artery walls that can affect blood vessels supplying the kidneys. The nerve and blood supply to the penis can also be damaged by diabetes, causing impotence.

What are the symptoms?

The first sign of kidney damage is the presence in urine of protein (proteinuria, p. 151). Patients are usually unaware of this, although it can be detected by dipstick tests. As proteinuria worsens, ankle swelling and symptoms of nephrotic syndrome may develop (p. 147). As diabetic nephropathy (kidney disease) advances, symptoms of uraemia (p. 154) and chronic renal failure (p. 145) may occur. End-stage renal failure may result, requiring dialysis or a kidney transplant. (Diabetic renovascular disease can also cause kidney failure and hypertension.)

How is it diagnosed?

Strictly, diabetic nephropathy can only be confirmed by renal biopsy (p. 105), but a biopsy is usually carried out only if additional factors suggest a kidney disorder. The condition is generally diagnosed from a patient's history and symptoms.

What are the treatment options?

Diabetes can be treated by insulin injection, tablets or by dietary modification, depending upon its severity. Studies have shown that the progress of diabetic nephropathy can be slowed by good diabetic control and by treating high blood pressure. ACE I and ACE II inhibitors are beneficial, and may even be useful in diabetic patients with normal blood pressure. Impotence can be treated by a variety of drugs. No treatment can reverse diabetic kidney disease, but transplantation of the insulin-producing cells of the pancreas may eventually offer a cure for some forms of diabetes.

GLOMERULONEPHRITIS

An inflammation of the glomerulus, the filtration unit of the kidney, caused by a wide variety of diseases.

The term glomerulonephritis (GN) refers to an unusual group of diseases that result in damage to the glomerulus. Some of these disorders are limited to the kidney, such as minimal change nephropathy, focal segmental glomerulosclerosis (FSGS), IgA nephropathy (p. 143) and membranous nephropathy. Others can also affect other organs and tissues, such as systemic lupus erythematosus (SLE) or Goodpasture's syndrome (p. 140). The risk of developing the various forms of GN is age dependent. Children are more likely to develop minimal change nephropathy and FSGS, adults IgA nephropathy, and the elderly membranous nephropathy.

What are the causes?

Most forms of GN are of unknown cause. It is probable that many are autoimmune in nature – in other words they result from the body's immune system mistakenly producing antibodies that attack, or become deposited in, the glomerulus. In some disorders, such as Goodpasture's syndrome, the specific abnormal antibody has been identified (p. 140). Some forms of GN are associated with infection, such as post-infectious GN.

What are the symptoms?

Most patients have haematuria (p. 140), proteinuria (p. 151) or kidney failure (p. 145), alone or in combination. Haematuria is not usually visible to the naked eye; severe proteinuria can cause nephritic syndrome (p. 134).

How is it diagnosed?

GN can usually only be diagnosed by kidney biopsy. This also allows the nephrologist and kidney pathologist to determine the specific type of GN affecting the kidney. In some forms of GN, such as Goodpasture's syndrome, blood tests are available to make the diagnosis (p. 100).

What are the treatment options?

In most forms of glomerulonephritis, the drugs that suppress the immune system, such as steroids, have been used as treatment, but this approach has not been universally successful and must be weighed against the potentially serious side effects of these drugs. Ingesting fish oils have also been shown to be beneficial in some studies, but this remains controversial. Blood pressure control is important because it helps to slow down progression of the disease.

What is the outlook?

Ten years after diagnosis, around 15 per cent of patients may have reached end-stage kidney failure and require dialysis or a kidney transplant. Patients who are most at risk of developing kidney failure are those who have a large amount of proteinuria, high blood pressure or chronic kidney failure when the disease is first diagnosed.

GOODPASTURE'S SYNDROME

Goodpasture's disease, or anti-glomerular basement membrane (anti-GBM) disease, is a rare disorder in which harmful antibodies can be measured in the blood of patients who develop acute kidney failure.

What are the causes?

The antibodies are autoantibodies – they are produced by the individual's own white blood cells in order to attack other parts of the body. The body usually has a strict mechanism to control or abort the production of such antibodies. In the case of anti-GBM disease this mechanism fails and autoantibodies are produced, which attack the glomerular basement membrane within the kidney. This sparks off an inflammatory response that ultimately leads to the destruction of all the glomeruli and thus to kidney failure. Occasionally, patients describe small volumes of dark or blood-stained urine, which probably reflects the severity of the inflammation within the kidney tissue. A typical patient might visit the GP having noticed that he/she is passing less urine than usual and beginning to feel tired and perhaps nauseous. The diagnosis of kidney failure is confirmed by blood tests.

How is it diagnosed?

One of the most characteristic features of this disease is the rapidity with which kidney failure can develop, often within days, occasionally even hours. It is often associated with simultaneous haemorrhage into the lungs (pulmonary haemorrhage). In most patients this causes the coughing up of blood but some have silent bleeding into the alveoli and the bleeding might only be suspected if the patient is unduly breathless or has a low blood count or signs of lung haemorrhage on a chest X-ray.

The antibody binds to its target antigen within the basement membrane and initiates inflammation and injury. Males born with Alport's syndrome (p. 135) are known to lack the Goodpasture antigen either entirely or partially. These boys develop kidney failure in their late teens or early 20s and often suffer deafness and eye abnormalities.

Some experts have linked Goodpasture's disease to hydrocarbon exposure.

What are the treatment options?

Efforts are made to treat the condition by removing the circulating antibodies and preventing further production. It is essential that this is done as soon as possible if kidney function is to be salvaged and pulmonary haemorrhage stopped. Other interim measures to support breathing may be necessary but in general if dialysis is required to support the patient at the time of diagnosis there is little or no hope of recovering kidney function. If the patient in still producing urine, rapid removal of the autoantibody by plasma exchange and prevention of further antibody production by administering steroids and immunosupressants can be tried. Treatment is continued until all detectable antibodies have been removed and production has ceased. Kidney transplantation cannot be undertaken until the antibody has not been detected in the blood for at least 12 months.

HAEMATURIA

This term refers to the presence of blood in the urine, which is usually not visible to the eye.

A routine dipstick test for a range of possible conditions may reveal the presence of haematuria. Blood may enter the urine either from within the kidney, or it can be added to the urine after it has been formed. Because cancers of the urinary tract are an important cause of haematuria, a full investigation is always necessary.

How is it diagnosed?

The first investigation is an examination of the urine under a microscope to look for casts – clumps of red blood cells – and misshapen, damaged red cells. Both of these indicate that a patient has a glomerular disease and that blood is getting into the urine from within the kidney. In such circumstances, a kidney biopsy is often needed to define precisely what is going on. Normal-looking red cells and the absence of casts indicate that blood has been added to the urine after the urine has been produced. This may indicate an infection, kidney stones or cancer.

Most patients with haematuria have an ultrasound, abdominal X-ray and an intravenous urogram (p. 102). These images help to exclude tumours and stones. If the haematuria is coming from below the glomeruli and outside the kidney, a cystoscopy (p. 106) is necessary, and any bladder lesion can be biopsied. During the cystoscopy, tiny catheters can be inserted into the ureter and X-ray contrast fluid injected back up into the kidney to show the structure of the ureter and kidney. This can detect small tumours within the urinary collecting system. With modern cystoscopic techniques it is possible to look right up the ureters and into the renal pelvis of the kidney. Brushings and biopsies of any suspicious lesion can be taken. If the haematuria are shown to be due to an inflamed or damaged glomerulus, a kidney biopsy may be required.

What are the treatment options?
If no underlying cause for the haematuria is found, no treatment is necessary, but the patient should be monitored regularly to ensure that a serious condition does not emerge. Infections or stones can be treated; if the haematuria is caused by cancer, treatment will be aimed at eradicating the cancer, or improving quality of life if the cancer has progressed too far for hope of a cure.

HAEMOLYTIC URAEMIC SYNDROME
A potentially life-threatening cause of acute kidney failure that can result from food poisoning.

In recent years haemolytic uraemic syndrome (HUS) has hit the headlines as a result of several high-profile outbreaks of food poisoning. HUS is so called because its features include anaemia, due to the destruction of red blood cells (haemolysis), and acute renal failure. If severe, many organs are affected and death can occur through circulatory failure.

What are the causes?
The most widely recognised cause of HUS is infection by strain 0157 of the bacterium *Escherichia coli* (*E. coli* 0157). This bacterium is normally found in the digestive system of animals such as cattle and sheep, but it can infect humans through ingestion of undercooked or poorly reheated meat products and unwashed vegetables. Some cases of HUS have also followed direct handling of farm animals. The bacterium is believed to produce a toxin that damages the lining of blood vessels. This causes the destruction of blood cells travelling through the vessels, and also disrupts the blood supply to organs such as the kidneys.

HUS can also occur in the absence of *E.coli* infection – in these circumstances the cause is less clear. Certain drugs and some cancers have been associated with its development.

What are the symptoms?
In HUS associated with *E. coli* 0157, diarrhoea usually occurs around a week before the disease's onset. Symptoms include acute renal failure (p. 145), anaemia and sometimes bruising. The brain may be affected, leading to fits and coma, or the heart, resulting in heart failure.

How is it diagnosed?
A diagnosis can be confirmed by identifying broken-up red blood cells (schistocytes) in the blood. These result from cells passing through damaged blood vessels. The level of platelets – the blood cells responsible for clotting – is also low. In around half the cases associated with diarrhoea, *E. coli* 0157 can be isolated from the patient's faeces.

What are the treatment options?
The effects of HUS can be reduced by a fresh frozen plasma (FFP) transfusion, or a process called plasma exchange, in which plasma is removed from the patient's blood and replaced by FFP. Acute renal failure must be treated by dialysis. Affected individuals also receive treatment to support organs that are failing. Usually there is no advantage in treating the *E. coli* infection with antibiotics.

How can it be prevented or minimised?
The risk of food poisoning by *E. coli* 0157 can be minimised by making sure that meat is thoroughly cooked. Following contact with farm animals, hands should be washed carefully.

HENOCH-SCHONLEIN PURPURA (HSP)
HSP is a rare multi-system disorder, which usually affects children but can occasionally occur in adults.

Half of the children affected by HSP are under five years old, with boys twice as likely to get it as girls.

What are the symptoms?

HSP is characterised by the combination of a purpuric or petechial rash (small raised blood blisters) usually at points of pressure such as the buttocks and thighs, accompanied by haematuria (blood in the urine). This may be macroscopic (visible to the naked eye) or microscopic (only detectable by dipstick testing or microscopy of the urine). Large amounts of protein may also be present in the urine and many patients are nephrotic (p. 147). In addition, affected children usually develop pain in the abdomen and swollen joints, most commonly, elbows, knees, wrists and ankles. The abdominal pain is usually related to gut involvement in the disease process. Endoscopy may show the same purpuric lesions present on the skin on the bowel wall.

Rarely, one of these lesions can act as the starting point for the bowel to fold in upon itself. This complication, known as intussusception, is usually suspected when a child has unusually severe abdominal pain and there are signs of bowel obstruction. A sausage-like mass can be felt when the abdomen is examined and there is often blood in the child's stool. If this complication is not too far advanced, it is usually possible to push the involuting bowel back by introducing barium via an enema. Sometimes surgical correction is required.

The function of the kidneys is not necessarily impaired, although rarely patients need dialysis until such time as the kidneys recover. Very few patients develop progressive chronic renal failure.

How is it diagnosed?

A kidney biopsy reveals deposits of an immunoglobin protein (IgA) in the glomeruli. The IgA can also be seen in skin biopsies and occasionally there are elevated levels of IgA circulating in the blood.

The cause of HSP is unknown but relapses often follow sore throats; exposure to drugs and to the cold have also been implicated in this disorder. There are similarities between the nephritis of HSP and IgA nephropathy (p. 143). Both conditions can recur following a kidney transplant.

What are the treatment options?

Treatment of this condition is usually with oral corticosteroids and – rarely – immunosuppressants, which shorten the duration of the attack. In some patients the episodes resolve spontaneously. Recurrent attacks are common and although, in general, the frequency and severity of attacks diminish as the child grows older, some individuals are dogged with attacks well into adult life.

HYDRONEPHROSIS

This is the distension of the renal calyces and the pelvis of the kidney, caused by an obstruction to the flow of urine.

What are the causes?

The renal calyces and renal pelvis act like a system of funnels, collecting urine from the different parts of the kidney and channelling it into the top of the ureter so that it can run down to the bladder and out of the body.

A blockage anywhere along the urinary tract will lead to back pressure and distension of the calyces and pelvis. The site of the obstruction determines whether one or both kidneys are affected. An obstruction to the outflow of urine in the bladder or urethra, such as an enlarged prostate, will affect both kidneys. If the obstruction is higher up in one or other ureter, it will affect only the kidney on that side. Causes of obstruction include stones, tumours of the urinary tract, scar tissue, prostatic enlargement and tumours close to some part of the urinary tract that cause compression.

What are the symptoms?

Often there are no symptoms initially, especially if the hydronephrosis develops slowly. If the obstruction is complete, hydronephrosis develops quickly and backache is common. The pain is made worse by drinking large amounts

---

AT THE LEADING EDGE

In utero imaging of hydronephrosis

Developments in ultrasound techniques now mean that, in skilled hands, the kidneys of an unborn baby can be seen on a scan by 17 weeks and potential problems with kidney function, including hydronephrosis, identified early. Happily, four out of five fetuses diagnosed with a problem through ultrasound will achieve normal kidney function by the end of the pregnancy or by the end of the baby's first year. Hydronephrosis in one kidney does not warrant intervention in utero. If the condition is present in both kidneys, intervention may occasionally be considered necessary. This might involve aspirating the fetus's urine to remove it, or inserting a shunt to improve urine flow. These procedures are carried out in a very few specialist centres. In most cases, the preferred management method is ultrasound soon after birth, followed by standard tests of kidney function.

of water or alcohol. There may be other symptoms related to the cause of the hydronephrosis, such as haematuria (blood in the urine), if a tumour is the cause of obstruction.

How is it diagnosed?
A diagnosis of hydronephrosis should always be considered in anyone with obstructive urinary symptoms, such as poor flow rate and having to strain to empty the bladder. A physical examination is helpful, since the kidneys may be enlarged and tender. The diagnosis is confirmed with an intravenous urogram (IVU) or an ultrasound scan.

What are the treatment options?
Treatment consists of identifying the cause of the obstruction and clearing it. This may involve removing a stone that is blocking a ureter, or a transurethral resection of the prostate (p. 130). If the kidneys are severely affected, and a rapid solution is necessary to allow urine to drain, a nephrostomy tube may be temporarily inserted through the skin into the renal pelvis to allow urine to drain while a permanent solution to the obstruction is planned.

How can it be prevented or minimised?
The consequences of hydronephrosis are minimised by early detection, before permanent kidney damage occurs. It should therefore always be considered as a possibility in any patient with a disorder that could lead to obstruction of a ureter, the bladder neck or urethra. This is one reason why intravenous urograms and ultrasound scans are common in urology.

IGA NEPHROPATHY
The commonest form of glomerulonephritis in the developed world, in which some patients eventually develop chronic kidney failure.

IgA nephropathy is so called because immunoglobulin A (IgA), an antibody that the body produces to fight infection, becomes abnormally deposited in the filtration units of the kidney, the glomeruli. This may eventually prevent the filter from working properly and lead to the irreversible destruction of glomeruli.

What are the causes?
The cause of IgA nephropathy is not known. There is some evidence that it may result from an abnormal response to infection, but it may also be related to differences between individuals in the chemical make-up of their IgA.

What are the symptoms?
Haematuria (p. 140) and/or proteinuria (p. 151), often only detected by dipstick testing, are common. Sometimes patients see blood in their urine, often after a respiratory infection. Occasionally IgA nephropathy is detected when a patient is found to have chronic kidney failure. Some patients are troubled with intermittent loin pain, especially during respiratory infections.

How is it diagnosed?
IgA nephropathy can only be definitely diagnosed by a kidney biopsy (p. 105). Special stains are used to show up the IgA deposited in the glomerulus.

What are the treatment options?
Immunosuppressives (drugs that suppress the immune system, such as steroids) have been used as treatment, but this approach has not been universally successful and must be weighed against the potentially serious side effects of these drugs. Fish oils has also been shown to be beneficial in some clinical studies, but remains controversial. Blood pressure control is important because it helps to slow down progression of the disease.

What is the outlook?
Ten years after diagnosis, 15 per cent of patients may have end-stage kidney failure and require dialysis or a transplant. Patients most at risk of kidney failure are those who have a large amount of proteinuria, high blood pressure or chronic kidney failure when the disease is first diagnosed.

INCONTINENCE
Urinary incontinence is the involuntary leakage of urine from the bladder.

Incontinence is a widespread health problem affecting the physical, social and economic well-being of many individuals and their families. There are various types.
- **Stress incontinence** Increased pressure in the abdomen due to coughing, sneezing or exercise causes leakage.
- **Urge incontinence** This is the sudden feeling of desperately needing to pass urine and not being able to hold on until reaching the toilet.
- **Overflow incontinence** This occurs if the bladder does not empty efficiently and so fills beyond its normal capacity and leaks urine. A patient may not be aware that the bladder never fully empties, only that it leaks continuously.

What are the causes?

One of the significant features of this condition is that similar symptoms can have very different causes.

- **Stress incontinence** Leaking when a person coughs or sneezes is usually caused by a weakness in the bladder neck, due to a lack of support from the pelvic floor or from a weak sphincter muscle (intrinsic sphincter deficiency). However, in a small but significant number of people with incontinence (10–15 per cent), an overactive bladder causes these symptoms. As the treatments are different, it is important to establish the cause of the incontinence as a first step.
- **Urge incontinence** This is more common in women and is usually caused by an overactive bladder muscle, but may occasionally be part of a neurological condition.
- **Overflow incontinence** This can be caused by an obstruction to the outflow of urine from the bladder, such as an enlarged prostate gland. Another cause is weak bladder muscles that are not capable of generating enough pressure to empty the bladder; this may result from nerve damage, possibly caused by a spinal cord injury or diabetes.

What are the symptoms?

By definition, the main symptom is the involuntary leakage of urine from the bladder. It is useful to note in what circumstances the leaking occurs, for how long it has been going on, and how often it happens.

How is it diagnosed?

Although the diagnosis of incontinence is fairly obvious from the symptoms alone, it is a little more complicated to diagnose the type of incontinence and the mechanism responsible. A thorough medical history and physical examination will both give valuable clues as to the likely cause. The completion of a frequency volume chart allows the doctor to assess fluid input, bladder capacity, when episodes of leaking take place and how often. A midstream urine sample (MSU) is essential, since a urinary tract infection can make incontinence worse. If surgery is being considered to treat stress incontinence, urodynamic tests must be performed first. Surgery will not help those patients whose leakage is caused by an overactive bladder muscle rather than a weak bladder neck, and may make their symptoms worse.

Other investigations may be required, depending upon any other symptoms. For example, neurological tests may be necessary if there are symptoms of muscle weakness or

HELP YOUR DOCTOR TO HELP YOU

Describing incontinence

Many people are reluctant to seek help from their doctor for urinary incontinence, either because they are embarrassed by it or because they incorrectly believe it to be an inevitable part of growing older. This is not so, and much can be done to improve the symptoms for the 5–15 per cent of the population who various studies have shown to be affected by incontinence. There is no need to be embarrassed when describing your symptoms. Your doctor will be used to dealing with this condition and will be interested in your particular circumstances.

- *Describe how long you have had the symptoms, and whether there was anything which preceded the onset of leaking (such as the birth of a baby).*
- *Tell your doctor how often you leak and what activities cause it to happen.*
- *Do your symptoms impact on your social and sexual activities?*
- *A frequency volume chart will give your doctor an overview of your bladder function.*

loss of sensation. If overflow incontinence is suspected, the upper urinary tract will normally be investigated with an intravenous urogram (IVU) or ultrasound scan.

What are the treatment options?

There is a wide range of different treatments for incontinence. If a treatment is to be successful, it must be very specifically targeted towards the underlying cause of the urine leakage.

- **Stress incontinence** caused by a weak bladder neck (usually called genuine stress incontinence) is often improved by relatively simple measures such as pelvic floor physiotherapy, weight loss and stopping smoking. If these fail to control the symptoms adequately, a variety of operations exist to treat the condition (p. 121).
- **Urge incontinence** can be treated by anticholinergic drugs. A continence advisor can offer advice on changing drinking patterns and lifestyle in order to minimise the problem, and will supervise bladder training.

• **Overflow incontinence** treatment relies on ensuring that the bladder empties completely to prevent hydronephrosis (p. 142) and urinary tract infections, which will occur if stagnant urine is allowed to collect in the bladder. If the condition is caused by an outflow obstruction, removing the obstruction often solves the problem. However, if it is caused by weak bladder muscles, it is unlikely that normal bladder function will return and so the bladder must be emptied by a catheter.

How can it be prevented or minimised?
Although not much can be done to prevent this condition altogether, most forms of incontinence are improved by changes in lifestyle. Drinking excess fluid increases urine production, so more leaking occurs: 1.5 to 2 litres (2½ to 3¼ pints) a day should be sufficient liquid for most people. Alcohol, tea, coffee and cola irritate the bladder and make it more active, and so should be avoided.

KIDNEY CANCER
The eighth most common cancer in men and the tenth most common cancer in women.

There are three main types of kidney cancer. The most common type arises from the kidney itself and accounts for 85 per cent of all such cancers: this is renal cell carcinoma. Less commonly, cancer can arise from the lining of the urine-transporting tubes (transitional cell carcinoma) or can occur in children (Wilm's tumour).

What are the causes?
The cause is unknown but exposure to cigarette smoke, obesity and hypertension have all been implicated.

What are the symptoms?
As with all forms of cancer, symptoms may be due to:
• the effects of the primary tumour (blood in the urine or the presence of a detectable lump in the abdomen);
• secondary spread such as a fracture occurring in a bone weakened by a deposit of the tumour at that site;
• general signs of malignant disease, such as weight loss.

How is it diagnosed?
With the widespread availability of abdominal imaging by means of ultrasound CT and MRI scanning, many renal cancers are nowadays picked up as so-called 'incidental findings', often at an early stage.

What is the prognosis?
The extent of the spread of the cancer when it is diagnosed can profoundly affect the prognosis, with patients who are found to have disease localised in the kidney at that time having as much as a 95 per cent chance of surviving the next five years. If the cancer has spread locally (around the kidney), survival for five years falls to 65 per cent, whereas 80 per cent of those with distant spread (to the lungs or bones, for example) do not survive for two years.

What are the treatment options?
Surgical excision of the kidney and adjacent tissues (radical nephrectomy) is the treatment of choice for localised disease. There have been recent developments in the surgical management of particularly the smaller tumours, with partial removal of the kidney, radiofrequency ablation, cryotherapy and laparoscopic removal all being used for selected patients with encouraging results. The treatment of advanced kidney cancer, however, is more difficult as this is not generally amenable to the standard cancer therapies such as chemo and radiation therapy. Recent advances and developments in immunotherapy involving interleukin and stem cell transplantation are providing new hope for patients with advanced kidney cancer.

KIDNEY FAILURE
Failure of the kidneys may occur suddenly (acute renal failure) or insidiously (chronic renal failure).

The major consequences of both acute and chronic kidney failure are an accumulation of metabolic waste products in the bloodstream due to failure of the excretory function of the kidney and the development of other complications of kidney failure. These problems develop rapidly over a few days in a patient with acute kidney failure, but over several months or even years in chronic kidney failure. Acute kidney failure generally occurs in a patient who is already ill or who undergoes major surgery during which the blood supply (and therefore delivery of oxygen) to the kidneys is compromised.

What are the causes?
The most frequent causes of acute kidney failure are:
• severe infection;
• surgery to the heart or major blood vessels;
• serious liver disease;
• major injury;
• extensive burns.

In contrast, chronic kidney failure occurs in patients who already have a kidney disease that causes progressive damage to both organs. Such diseases might only damage the kidneys (such as glomerulonephritis, p. 139), or they may be more generalised (such as diabetes, p. 139). Occasionally, patients with chronic kidney failure develop a sudden decline in kidney function as a result of illness, so-called acute on chronic kidney failure.

How is it diagnosed?

Because acute kidney failure usually affects patients who are already very sick, it often occurs in hospital and is readily detected by routine blood tests that show a sudden and rapid rise in levels of urea and creatinine from a normal baseline, over a period of a few days.

In contrast, patients with chronic kidney failure may feel well, particularly in the early stages, and so can be unaware that they have kidney disease. The illness may be identified during blood tests taken for another reason. Such patients need further investigation to find out the cause of their kidney disease, so it can be treated to slow kidney damage. A small number of patients only consult a doctor at a late stage when symptoms of uraemia (p. 154) develop. In such cases, the kidneys are often already significantly damaged.

What are the treatment options?

Patients with either acute or chronic kidney failure may need dialysis to treat the life-threatening complications of uraemia. With acute kidney failure, assuming the patient survives the illness or operation that caused the kidneys to fail, kidney function is likely to recover, usually after a few weeks, and dialysis can then be ended. Full restoration of normal kidney function is usual in such patients. With patients who have chronic kidney failure – caused by long-term, progressive damage to both kidneys – recovery of kidney function does not occur, and if their kidneys deteriorate enough to require dialysis treatment, the dialysis is lifelong; the only alternative is a kidney transplant.

KIDNEY STONES

Stones form from the constituents of urine when the concentrations of substances that make up the stones rise too high and are no longer dissolved in urine.

About 15 per cent of Caucasian men and 6 per cent of Caucasian women suffer from a kidney stone at some point in their lives. Half experience a recurrence at a later date.

What are the causes?

Stones of differing composition have differing causes.
- **Calcium** Diet, excess calcium in the urine, excess vitamin A and D, prolonged immobility, overactive parathyroid glands, sarcoidosis, kidney acidification defect
- **Oxalate** Inherited metabolic disease, diet
- **Uric acid** Gout, rare inherited metabolic disorders
- **Triple phosphate** Infection, obstruction
- **Cystine** Inherited metabolic disease

Normal urine contains some elements that inhibit stone formation, such as magnesium, citrate and pyrophosphate, and some proteins produced within the kidney (nephrocalcin and Tamm-Horsfall protein) also retard stone formation. The acidity of the urine may also play a role: for example, calcium is more soluble in acid urine but uric acid is more soluble in an alkaline urine.

How are they diagnosed?

Investigation is required to identify the underlying causes of stone formation. Blood is taken to measure the levels of parathyroid hormone, vitamin D, calcium, phosphate, bicarbonate, chloride and uric acid. A 24-hour urine sample collection will be required to measure the daily excretion of sodium, calcium, phosphate, uric acid, oxalate and citrate. Urine will be sent for culture to exclude an infection. Tests may be required to look for more subtle abnormalities such as the inability to make an acid urine.

Most calculi contain calcium and are therefore opaque to X-rays and can be easily identified. Cystine stones (made of a sulphur-containing amino acid) are also radio-opaque but uric acid stones are radiolucent and therefore more difficult to demonstrate. It is thought that tiny crystals of uric acid may form a seed around which calcium stones then form.

What are the treatment options?

Treatment depends on the nature of the minerals forming the stones, as well as any underlying metabolic cause. The most important aspect of treatment is to increase the amount of urine produced so that the concentration of the dissolved minerals is kept low. This may mean the patient drinking at least 3 litres (5¼ pints) of water each day. It is important that this water is not high in calcium or sodium.

Potassium citrate can be given (450mg, 2–3 times a day) to retard urinary crystal and stone growth and to make the urine more alkaline, which slows the precipitation of uric acid. Diet plays an important role in reducing the risk of stone formation. A diet rich in calcium, vitamin D, sodium or protein should be modified. Paradoxically, however, a very low calcium diet is counterproductive because dietary calcium binds to dietary oxalate, preventing the absorption of the oxalate from the intestine. A low-calcium diet, therefore, allows more oxalate to be absorbed, raising blood and urine oxalate and increasing the risk of oxalate stones. Most doctors now advise a calcium intake of about 1000 mmol per day in patients who form these stones.

A high excretion of calcium in the urine can be reduced by taking low doses of one of the thiazide diuretics such as bendrofluazide or indapamide.

The nature, size and site – kidney, bladder or ureter – of the stone decide the best surgical approach to treatment. Treatment of stones in the kidney has been revolutionised by the development of extracorporeal shock wave lithotripsy (ESWL, p. 119). Alternatively, a stone in the bladder or a ureter can be directly fragmented following cystoscopy (p. 106) using a probe with ultrasound or a high-energy laser beam. Other approaches include passing a large tube directly into the kidney through the back (a nephrostomy tube) and passing instruments through the tube to break up the stone (p. 120).

What is the outlook?

Patients with recurrent stone episodes should be referred for investigation so that measures can be taken to reduce the risk of further stone formation.

NEPHRITIS

See Acute nephritis p. 134; Glomerulonephritis p. 139; Tubulo-interstitial nephritis, p. 153.

NEPHROTIC SYNDROME

A consequence of excess protein in the urine, nephrotic syndrome usually causes the ankles to swell.

Nephrotic syndrome is the combination of large quantities of protein in the urine (proteinuria), low albumin in the blood (hypoalbuminaemia) and tissue swelling (oedema). If kidneys leak too much protein into the urine (usually more than 3g per day, see proteinuria, p. 151), levels of albumin, a protein found in the blood, fall below normal. Albumin plays an important role in retaining fluid within blood vessels, so as it falls fluid leaks into the body's tissues. Because of gravity, this fluid accumulates first in the feet and lower legs, causing the ankles to swell.

What are the causes?

Any cause of heavy proteinuria may result in an individual becoming nephrotic. Common causes include diabetes and forms of glomerulonephritis (p. 139). There is a rare form of nephrotic syndrome that is present from birth (p. 137).

What are the symptoms?

Typically, the main symptom is tissue swelling of the feet and lower legs. If the blood albumin is very low, clots can develop within blood vessels and, very occasionally, cause a pulmonary embolus (a clot within the blood vessels of the lung). The cholesterol level in the blood can also increase.

What are the treatment options?

If possible, the underlying cause of the nephrotic syndrome should be treated. Oedema can be reduced by diuretics – drugs that increase the flow of urine. The proteinuria can be treated with ACE inhibitors, which have been shown to reduce the amount of protein excreted in the urine. If the blood albumin is very low, it may be necessary to reduce the chances of blood clotting with drugs such as warfarin. High cholesterol can be treated by drugs known as statins.

NEUROPATHIC BLADDER

This term describes abnormal bladder function resulting from diseases that affect the nerves serving the bladder.

What are the causes?

Most neurological diseases that affect the spinal cord cause bladder dysfunction, as can some that affect the brain, including Parkinson's disease, spinal cord injuries and tumours of the central nervous system. Diseases that damage the peripheral nerves around the bladder, such as multiple sclerosis and diabetes, may also cause bladder dysfunction.

What are the symptoms?

These vary according to the type of neurological disease that is giving rise to the loss of normal bladder control. Often the bladder muscle is 'unstable' and contracts strongly without conscious control, causing incontinence. This is known as detrusor hyperreflexia and is frequently accompanied by detrusor sphincter dyssynergia (p. 138). Another symptom can be greatly diminished bladder muscle strength, resulting in inefficient bladder emptying. Alternatively or in addition, a patient can experience a complete loss of bladder sensation and so be no longer able to tell when the bladder is full and needs to be emptied.

How is it diagnosed?

Diagnosis is complex and requires the specialist skills of a neurologist. Often a diagnosis may be hinted at by clues in the medical history, such as other symptoms relating to the nervous system. There may also be findings from a physical examination, such as a loss of sensation, which point to a neurological cause. Videocystometrography is useful since it gives detailed information on the bladder and urethral function during the filling, storing and emptying phases. Specialist neurological tests then need to be performed, depending on what type of underlying disease is suspected.

What are the treatment options?

Treatment varies according to the nature of the neurological disease and the way in which it affects the bladder. If the bladder is 'unstable' because of detrusor hyperreflexia, anticholinergic drugs will help to stabilise it. If, however, the bladder is unable to contract because of damage to the nerve supply, it must be emptied by use of clean intermittent self-catheterisation (CISC) to prevent overflow incontinence and lasting damage to the kidneys. If this is not possible, a long-term suprapubic catheter may need to be inserted.

How can it be prevented or minimised?

There is little that can be done to prevent the neurological conditions that give rise to neuropathic bladder, but fortunately this is a rare cause of urinary disorders.

NOCTURNAL ENURESIS
The habitual, involuntary passage of urine at night, better known as bedwetting.

Bedwetting is common in childhood but becomes less common with age, with only 1 per cent of adults affected. If an individual has never had night-time control of the bladder since early childhood, the condition is termed primary nocturnal enuresis. If there has been a period of control followed by relapse, it is known as secondary enuresis.

What are the causes?

A small minority of individuals are shown to have a neurological problem or an abnormality of the urinary tract, but in most people no obvious cause is found. Many experts believe that nocturnal enuresis represents a delay in the maturation of the mechanisms that control continence.

About a quarter of four year olds regularly wet the bed.

What are the symptoms?

The main symptom by definition is bedwetting at night. Usually there are no other urinary symptoms. If other symptoms are present, such as urgency and frequency, it is more likely that there is another cause such as an overactive bladder or an infection.

How is it diagnosed?

The diagnosis is reached by excluding other causes. Where persistent bedwetting is the only symptom, urinalysis, a midstream urine sample (MSU) to look for infection and an ultrasound scan of the urinary tract are sufficient investigations. If there are other troublesome urinary symptoms, urodynamic tests may be indicated. None of these tests are usually performed on children.

What are the treatment options?

There are two approaches to treatment, which can be used together to good effect.
- **Behaviour modification** This takes the form of an enuresis alarm, which is triggered by detecting moisture on either the sheets or nightclothes, and wakes the individual. Gradually a person learns not to wet at night. It may take some time to show an improvement, but there is proven benefit in over 75 per cent of cases. This method can be used for both children and adults.
- **Drug treatment** The drug DDAVP (desmopressin acetate), a man-made version of the natural hormone vasopressin, reduces urine production. If taken before bed, DDAVP reduces bladder filling overnight, making bedwetting less likely. Tricyclic antidepressants can also be effective (p. 109). They have an antispasmodic action on the bladder, which makes it less likely that the bladder will unconsciously contract.

How can it be prevented or minimised?

The likelihood of nocturnal enuresis can be minimised by not drinking excessive amounts of fluid in the evening and avoiding caffeine in drinks such as tea, coffee and cola.

OEDEMA
The retention of salt and water in the body.

Excess fluid collects outside the tissues and cells and also outside the blood compartment, and occupies the spaces between the cells of the body – the so-called interstitial space. If sufficient fluid accumulates, it is noticeable as swelling and can be demonstrated as an indentation in the tissues following firm pressure with a finger. Oedema collects at the lowest parts of the body; when a person is standing the ankles and legs swell, when lying in bed, the back and sacral areas swell. To be detected by pressure, at least 5 litres (1 gallon) of excess fluid has been retained.

What are the causes?

Oedema fluid forms as a result of an imbalance of the physical forces acting across the walls of the tiny blood vessels called capillaries. It is via the capillaries that oxygen, blood and nutrition are supplied to the tissues and organs of the body. The cells of the capillary wall are porous to allow the exchange of waste products produced by other cells for nutritional replenishment from the blood.

Normally, some fluid leaves the arterial end of the capillaries because of the high pressure generated by the pumping action of the heart. This fluid (called interstitial fluid) bathes the tissue cells, which enables a free interchange of nutrition and waste products, then returns to the circulation via a system of tiny drainage channels known as the lymphatics. Some interstitial fluid is sucked back into the capillaries near the small veins because the blood pressure at the venous end of the capillaries is much lower than at the arterial end. Most of the salt and water in the bloodstream is retained inside the blood vessels and capillaries because of a sucking action exerted by high concentrations of proteins that are too big to leak out of the capillary wall. The most important protein for this action is albumin. The tendency of proteins in the bloodstream to retain fluid within the circulatory space is known as the plasma oncotic pressure. Oedema is caused by a malfunction of this process, and may form for any one of a variety of reasons.

- **Higher than normal blood pressure at the arterial end of the capillaries** – possibly caused by medications to regulate high blood pressure, which dilate the small arteries.
- **Leaky capillary walls** – due to physical damage such as irradiation, sunburn, or burns and scalds; allergy; scurvy; or severe infection such as septicaemia.
- **Low oncotic pressure in the blood** – caused by low protein concentration in the blood, for example in patients with heavy proteinuria (p. 151) or who are malnourished; liver disease may cause loss of oncotic pressure.
- **Higher than normal blood pressure at the venous end of the capillary** – main causes are heart failure or thrombosis.
- **Failure of the lymphatic circulation** – caused by prolonged standing or immobility, and by blockage of the lymphatics due to tumours, infections or external pressure.

Oedema may lead to heaviness in the lower limbs. It is not in itself dangerous, but often a sign of serious kidney, heart or liver disease, requiring full investigation.

What are the treatment options?

Treatment depends on the main cause. A reduction in salt and water intake can help to reduce oedema. Avoiding long periods of standing and raising the legs when sitting may also help. Wearing firm, full-length compression stockings or tights helps to keep fluid within the circulation and improves the return of venous blood and lymph to the heart and circulation. Diuretics can be used, with care, to encourage the kidneys to eliminate more salt and water via the urine. Occasionally, it may be necessary to increase the protein (albumin) concentration of the blood by giving intravenous human albumin solutions. Much can be done to prevent and control oedema by the proper medical management of underlying kidney, heart or liver disease.

OVERACTIVE BLADDER
This is a condition in which the bladder contracts even though the person is trying to stop it from doing so.

An alternative medical name for the condition is detrusor instability. It is more common in women than in men.

What are the causes?

In most cases this is a disorder that a person is born with and may get better or worse depending on other factors. There is no specific cause and no neurological problem, and the functioning of the kidneys and urinary tract is otherwise normal. Less often, bladder overactivity is a result of some disease or disorder, such as an enlarged prostate in men. It can also happen in women as a result of surgery for stress incontinence.

An overactive bladder regularly occurs in as much as 10 per cent of the population.

What are the symptoms?

Typical symptoms are a frequent need and urgency to urinate, nocturia (having to get up to urinate at night) and, in some cases, urge incontinence (p. 143).

How is it diagnosed?

Diagnosis will be strongly suspected from the symptoms. A frequency volume chart showing small volumes of urine passed frequently throughout the day and often at night also point toward the diagnosis. It can be confirmed through urodynamic tests (p. 101), which will usually show a rise in pressure (indicating the presence of bladder muscle contractions) while the bladder is being filled or 'provoked' by the patient listening to running water. These muscle contractions occur even while the patient is making an active attempt to stop them.

What are the treatment options?

The most effective treatment is a combination of bladder training with a continence advisor and drug therapy with anticholinergic drugs (p. 108). This will improve symptoms in over 90 per cent of cases if the treatment is properly followed. There is a wide range of anticholinergic drugs: it may require some testing to find the most appropriate for each patient. In the few cases where treatment does not work after a reasonable trial, it is possible to instil strong solutions of anticholinergic drugs directly into the bladder. If this fails, either neuromodulation (p. 112) or a clam cystoplasty (p. 129) may be considered.

How can it be prevented or minimised?

In most cases, little can be done to prevent this condition, unless it is a secondary result of an obstruction. The effects can be minimised, however, by lifestyle changes. Drinking excessive amounts of fluid exacerbates the symptoms: 1.5 to 2 litres (2½ to 3½ pints) per day should be sufficient for most people. Alcohol, tea, coffee and cola act as diuretics, leading to increased urinary frequency, and irritate the bladder, making it even more active. For these reasons, these beverages are best avoided.

POLYCYSTIC KIDNEY DISEASE (PKD)
The commonest form of inherited kidney disease, this condition often causes kidney failure in late middle age.

Autosomal dominant polycystic kidney disease (ADPKD) is an inherited disorder that affects around 1 in 500 people. It is characterised by the development of cysts within the kidneys. These increase in size and number during an individual's life, causing the kidneys to enlarge and – eventually – to fail.

What are the causes?

Most cases of polycystic kidney disease are caused by a mutation in the gene polycystin 1. (A few cases are caused by mutations in a related gene, polycystin 2.) Everyone inherits two copies of the polycystin 1 gene, one from their father and one from their mother. Only one copy needs to be mutated to cause polycystic kidney disease – this pattern of inheritance is described as autosomal dominant. This means that children of an individual with polycystic kidney disease have a one in two chance of developing the disease themselves. A rarer form of polycystic kidney disease, autosomal recessive polycystic disease, also exists, which typically causes kidney failure in childhood.

What are the symptoms?

Because the kidney cysts enlarge very slowly, there are often no early symptoms. Occasionally, blood can be seen in the urine. If the kidneys become very large, they can cause abdominal discomfort. Sometimes bleeding occurs within a cyst, resulting in acute pain. If cysts become infected, abdominal pain can be accompanied by fever. Stones form in about 30 per cent of patients; these, too, can cause pain.

PKD affects 12.5 million people around the world, more than cystic fibrosis, muscular dystrophy, haemophilia, Down's syndrome and sickle cell anaemia combined.

As the kidneys fail, high blood pressure and uraemia develop (p. 154). Cysts can also occur in other organs, such as the liver and pancreas, but these usually do not cause symptoms. Some people with polycystic kidney disease develop swelling in blood vessels in the brain – these can bleed causing subarachnoid haemorrhage, a form of stroke.

How is it diagnosed?

Cysts are typically detected by ultrasound, CT scanning or by MRI. A positive diagnosis can usually be made in early adulthood, but it can be difficult to rule out ADPKD in children, when cysts are in the early stages of development. Because of this, and because there is no specific treatment for early polycystic kidney disease, most nephrologists do not recommend screening the children of affected individuals until they are adult.

What are the treatment options?

There is no specific treatment for polycystic kidney disease. Complications such as high blood pressure and infection should be treated if they develop. As the kidneys fail, uraemia is treated and dialysis started. Kidney transplantation is usually possible. It is unusual to have to remove a polycystic kidney, but this is sometimes done if the kidney causes chronic pain or if the patient suffers from persistent kidney infections.

PROSTATITIS
An inflammation of the prostate gland in men, usually due to a bacterial infection.

Prostatitis is commonly associated with infections elsewhere, especially with urinary tract infections or sexually transmitted infections. It is found in all age groups, although the type of infection responsible usually changes with age. If the infection is not treated, it can progress to chronic prostatitis and result in long-term symptoms.

What are the causes?
The cause in young men is often a sexually transmitted infection, such as gonorrhoea. This ascends up the urethra to the prostate. The other major routes of infection are from urine or via the bloodstream.

What are the symptoms?
Symptoms typically start suddenly and include severe pain in the region of the prostate, lower back pain, a burning sensation on passing urine and sometimes passing blood in the urine, as well as fever and feeling run down.

How is it diagnosed?
The symptoms prompt a doctor to perform a rectal examination. This usually reveals a tender, swollen, warm prostate gland. Often the lymph nodes in the groin will also be swollen and tender. A midstream urine specimen (MSU) will usually be found to contain bacteria when examined under the microscope. By culturing the bacteria in the MSU sample it is possible to identify the type responsible, although results can take several days.

What are the treatment options?
The mainstay of treatment is antibiotic medication. This is normally started immediately, before the results of the MSU culture are available. If necessary, the antibiotics can be modified after a few days. Painkillers such as paracetamol are of benefit, and it is important to drink plenty of fluids. Constipation will exacerbate the pain and so laxatives are prescribed if this is a problem.

How can it be prevented or minimised?
The use of barrier contraception during sexual intercourse reduces the chances of developing prostatitis by the sexual route. Prompt investigation and treatment of suspected urinary tract infections decreases the risk of developing not only prostatitis but also acute pyelonephritis (p. 134).

PROTEINURIA
Excess protein in the urine.

Proteins are large molecules found within the fluid part of the blood, the plasma. Examples of proteins include antibodies, clotting factors and albumin. Urine is formed by the filtration of blood through the kidneys' many tiny filters, the glomeruli. These filters normally allow into the urine a very small quantity of protein (mostly albumin) and no blood cells at all. In normal circumstances, most people make about 1 litre of urine per day, which contains less than 50mg of protein. The presence of excess levels of protein in the urine may be an important marker of significant disease.

How is it diagnosed?
Proteinuria can be detected by simple dipstick tests or, more accurately, by chemical tests on the urine.

A level of protein in the urine that exceeds 50mg per day or per litre of urine is generally taken as an early warning of kidney disease, particularly in a patient who already has high blood pressure or diabetes.

However, there are instances when a reading of as much as 2000mg of protein in the urine is taken, but there is no serious underlying disease or disorder. This condition is called asymptomatic proteinuria and is benign. It is also known that proteinuria increases when we stand up. This is thought to be due to the kidneys moving forwards and down when we are upright, which slightly impairs the free drainage of blood from the kidneys, causing an increase in protein in the urine.

If protein in the urine exceeds 2000mg a day, there is usually a significant underlying cause that involves the kidneys in some way. Once proteinuria is in excess of 3000mg per day, the term 'nephrotic syndrome' is usually applied. Proteinuria of this magnitude generally exceeds the capacity of the liver to replace the proteins that are lost in the urine; as a result, oedema typically develops (p. 148).

What are the causes?
Causes of proteinuria include diabetes (p. 139), amyloidosis, glomerulonephritis (p. 139), high blood pressure, tubulo-interstitial nephritis (p. 153) and heart disease.

What are the treatment options?
Treatment should clearly be directed to the principal causes of proteinuria, but it is also important to try to reduce the amount of protein in the urine in its own right. This can be

done through blood-pressure lowering medication, such as ACE inhibitors and angiotensin receptor blocking drugs, which can reduce the blood pressure in the glomeruli as well as in the rest of the body.

What is the outlook?

The outlook is good for people whose proteinuria is caught early and controlled. Those with untreated proteinuria, however, run a significant risk of kidney failure.

REFLUX NEPHROPATHY

This condition is the result of the backward movement of urine when the bladder contracts.

Although often referred to as chronic pyelonephritis, reflux nephropathy is the more accurate term since, unlike acute pyelonephritis (p. 134), chronic pyelonephritis is not due to continuing infection, but is associated with sterile urine and does not respond to antibiotics.

What are the causes?

Reflux nephropathy is caused by the backward movement of urine (reflux), often under pressure, particularly if the bladder is abnormal. The condition arises during infancy and is associated with infection. The backward pressure and infection set up a process of inflammation and scarring in the kidney. Almost all the damage occurs in the first few years of life; new kidney scars are rare after the age of five.

How is it diagnosed?

Early detection and treatment of urine infection in infants can limit or prevent the development of scars in the kidney. Very young children cannot complain of the symptoms of a urinary tract infection and so the diagnosis can be missed. Infants fail to thrive, go off their food, and may have a fever without obvious kidney problems. In such circumstances the urine should always be cultured to check for infection.

What are the treatment options?

Until recently a substantial body of medical opinion felt that surgery should be performed to prevent the reflux of urine from the bladder up to the kidney. It is known, however, that reflux is very common in infants and usually resolves, particularly if infection is eradicated. Trials of surgery compared with antibiotics have not shown any benefit to surgery. If a child is at risk of reflux nephropathy because of persistent infection, long-term low-dose antibiotics are

usually indicated, until the kidney has finished growing. Every attempt should be made to keep the child free of infection, and any breakthrough infections while the child is on low-dose antibiotics should be vigorously treated.

What is the outlook?

The consequences of reflux during infancy vary from no symptoms at all to end-stage chronic renal failure. The scars may be small and only affect one kidney. A kidney scar can cause high blood pressure later in life, particularly during pregnancy. If, however, the scars affect both kidneys and are extensive, the patient may develop kidney failure in adult life and require dialysis or transplantation. The most common complication of reflux nephropathy is high blood pressure. This should be looked for and promptly treated. Evidence suggests that good control of blood pressure can significantly reduce the risk of progressive kidney failure.

RENAL ABSCESS

An infective abscess within the kidney.

This was more common before antibiotics were routinely available to treat infections. If an infection of any part of the body develops unchecked, bacteria will multiply and circulate in the blood. This is known as septicaemia. The bacteria are then carried to the kidneys, where clusters of them are deposited and establish a series of small abscesses. These later coalesce to form a larger inflammatory mass.

What are the causes?

The major causes are conditions that predispose to blood-borne infections. Vulnerable groups include poorly treated diabetics, drug takers who use infected equipment, and people with immune deficiencies, such as AIDS patients.

What are the symptoms?

The symptoms are pain in the back over the affected kidney, feeling unwell and fluctuating body temperature. This may be associated with rigor – coldness accompanied by shivering, followed by a hot sensation and sweating. If the abscess is not treated, the collection of pus will work its way to the surface and discharge through the skin.

How is it diagnosed?

The symptoms strongly suggest an infective process at work in the body. The first step is to try to find the focus of the infection. A physical examination is likely to reveal an enlarged kidney that is extremely tender to the touch. Microscopy of the urine may reveal the presence of pus cells, and an X-ray or ultrasound scan will show a mass within the affected kidney. By using ultrasound to guide a biopsy needle, some pus can be drawn off and analysed to see what sort of infection has caused the abscess.

What are the treatment options?

The modern treatment for this condition is high doses of intravenous antibiotics until the symptoms are controlled. If the response to antibiotics is poor, or if the abscess is particularly large, it may need to be drained surgically.

How can it be prevented or minimised?

Renal abscess is preventable in most people by ensuring that bacterial infections do not get out of control. This is can be done by prompt treatment with antibiotics. It is important to minimise the development of this condition, which leaves the kidney scarred and functioning poorly.

RETROGRADE EJACULATION

The passage of semen back into the bladder from the testes, rather than out along the male urethra.

What are the causes?

This occurs as a side effect of prostate surgery. It is not harmful, but anyone considering a transurethral resection of the prostate should be warned that there is a 70–80 per cent chance of this resulting. It is caused by damage to the normal valve mechanism at the neck of the bladder.

What are the symptoms?

The only symptom is not ejaculating semen from the end of the penile urethra at orgasm. Sexual desire, erectile function and orgasm are not affected by retrograde ejaculation itself. However, impotence can result from prostate surgery in 10–15 per cent of cases.

How is it diagnosed?

The diagnosis is evident – no investigations are necessary.

What are the treatment options?

This condition is not treatable, so patients must understand that it is likely to occur following prostate surgery. Most men who are counselled about the risk accept it, knowing that quality of life and sexual function are likely to improve as a result of the surgery. The desire to father more children is not usually an issue in the age group of men who undergo prostate surgery. If it is, however, semen can be extracted from the testes directly or filtered from the urine.

How can it be prevented or minimised?

Retrograde ejaculation is preventable by not undergoing surgery, but the benefits of prostate surgery in men with distressing urinary symptoms outweigh this consideration.

TUBULO-INTERSTITIAL NEPHRITIS

A destructive inflammatory process within the kidney.

The disease process spares the glomeruli but damages the tiny renal tubules that collect urine and pass it to the renal pelvis. There are acute and chronic types of the condition.

What are the causes?

- **Acute nephritis** Infection, toxins, autoimmune disorders
- **Chronic nephritis** Toxins such as Chinese herbs, infections such as tuberculosis, the inflammatory disorder sarcoidosis

The most common cause of both types of nephritis is an allergic reaction to one of many common drugs.

- **Acute** Antibiotics, non-steroidal anti-inflammatory drugs, allouinol, diuretics, phenytoin, omerprazole
- **Chronic** Lithium, mesalazine, cyclosporine, nitrosoureas, tacrolimus, some herbal medicines

How is it diagnosed?

Patients may initially suffer from a skin rash and fever. The urine usually contains blood and protein. Kidney function can deteriorate quite rapidly, with rising levels of urea and creatinine. Examination of the urine may show red blood cells, casts and the type of white blood cells known as eosinophils. A definitive diagnosis can be made by kidney biopsy. In rare cases, autoimmune disease can be associated with interstitial nephritis.

What are the treatment options?

Treatment involves the cessation of any offending drug and the eradication of any infection. Sometimes a short course of steroids can be helpful.

What is the outlook?

Provided acute inflammation is eradicated and there is no scarring, the prognosis is good. However, in cases involving chronic interstitial nephritis and marked scarring the likely outcome is slow progress toward chronic renal failure.

URAEMIA
The full spectrum of metabolic disorders that occur as a consequence of kidney failure.

Uraemia includes accumulation in the bloodstream of urea, a waste product of protein breakdown. Although urea is the most readily recognised 'uraemic toxin', a number of other breakdown products are also retained due to the inability of failing kidneys to eliminate them. Of these, levels of creatinine, a by-product of muscle metabolism, are often used as a measure of the severity of kidney failure. Potassium accumulation is especially dangerous because it can disturb the heart rhythm, leading to cardiac arrest. Elevated levels of phosphate contribute to the development of bone disease.

Uraemia is usually associated with the development of anaemia, caused by a deficiency of haemoglobin. While other conditions such as a lack of iron may cause anaemia in otherwise healthy individuals, in patients with kidney failure, anaemia is due to a deficiency of the hormone erythropoietin. Produced by the kidney, this stimulates the bone marrow to manufacture red cells that carry the haemoglobin round the body.

Many patients with uraemia develop symptoms of tiredness, loss of appetite, breathlessness and nausea.

What are the treatment options?
Symptoms can be corrected by dialysis and by medication. Erythropoietin can be produced synthetically and given by injection to correct the deficiency. A transplant may be an option in some cases.

URINARY TRACT INFECTION
A urinary tract infection (UTI) is a bacterial infection of some part of the urinary tract.

The affected part is usually the bladder and urethra, as in cystitis, but the upper urinary tract and kidneys may also be involved, when the condition is known as pyelonephritis. Urinary tract infection is a very common condition. It is more common in women, at least half of whom will suffer from a UTI during their lifetime. It is much less common in young men, but the incidence of UTI starts to increase in men over the age of 50. Repeated episodes that return despite treatment are called recurrent UTIs.

Up to 3 per cent of all GP consultations in the UK are for urinary tract infections. UTIs respond to antibiotics.

What are the causes?
Commonly the cause is bacteria entering the bladder via the urethra from the outside. This is termed an ascending infection. Sometimes bacteria are carried in the bloodstream to the urinary tract. Any condition that results in the bladder not emptying completely will make UTI more likely, as this results in stagnant urine collecting in the bladder. Predisposing disorders include obstruction such as benign prostatic hypertrophy (p. 135), ineffective bladder emptying, and neuropathic bladder disorders. Diabetes (p. 139) is a risk factor since bacteria thrive and multiply in sugary urine.

Recurrent urinary tract infections are caused by conditions that encourage the bacteria to reinfect the urinary tract. This includes congenital abnormalities, kidney stones and vesicoureteric reflux (p. 155).

What are the symptoms?
The classical symptoms are pain on passing urine, a frequent need and urge to pass urine, and nocturia. Often the urine appears cloudy and smells offensive. If the infection ascends the ureters, backache and fever may result. In the elderly, symptoms may include confusion and appetite loss.

How is it diagnosed?
A diagnosis is made on the basis of symptoms and urinalysis. In the presence of an infection, nitrates and white blood cells are typically detected in the urine. The definitive investigation is a midstream urine sample (MSU), which reveals the type of bacteria causing the infection and the most appropriate antibiotic; results are available in three days. Recurrent UTIs need more thorough investigation to establish the reason for the continued presence of bacteria in the urinary tract. This usually involves cystoscopy (p. 106) and an intravenous urogram (IVU) or ultrasound scan.

What are the treatment options?
Treatment is with antibiotics. These can be started at once if the symptoms are severe and urinalysis is positive, then adjusted once the results of the MSU are available. Usually 3–5 days' treatment is sufficient in women; men may need a longer course. In addition, 'flushing out' the urinary tract by drinking plenty of fluids is sometimes recommended.

How can it be prevented or minimised?
Passing urine after sex and drinking cranberry juice are often effective in preventing UTI. Treatment of any disorder that predisposes to infection, such as an obstructed bladder neck, will help to prevent future infections.

URINARY RETENTION
Inability to empty the bladder, leading to the bladder becoming stretched and enlarged.

There are two forms of urinary retention: acute, which s sudden, and chronic, which develops slowly over time.

What are the causes?
Three categories of conditions can cause urinary retention.
- Obstructions in the bladder neck and urethra such as stones, blood clots, an enlarged prostate or tumours.
- Obstructions compressing or kinking the urethra such as a pregnant uterus, fibroids or severe constipation.
- Disorders of the nerve supply to the bladder such that the bladder cannot contract strongly enough to expel urine.

What are the symptoms?
Symptoms depend on how quickly the bladder becomes distended. Acute urinary retention is painful and feels like a strong urge to pass urine, without being able to. Chronic retention builds slowly, so the bladder gets used to its larger capacity and there is no pain. There may be symptoms of the disorder that is causing the retention, such as poor flow and frequency caused by benign prostatic hypertrophy (p. 135).

How is it diagnosed?
The symptoms suggest the diagnosis, which can be confirmed by abdominal examination. This will reveal an enlarged bladder in the lower abdomen; the bladder can only be felt in this way when it is abnormally distended. Having made the diagnosis, it is important to consider the possible causes.

What are the treatment options?
Continued enlargement of the bladder is ended by inserting a catheter to enable it to drain properly. Over-stretching the bladder muscle leaves it weakened and unable to contract properly. If the bladder is allowed to rest whilst urine is drained through a catheter, it often regains some contractile function; however, a significant number of people never regain normal function if the bladder has been over-stretched.

How can it be prevented or minimised?
Urinary retention is often preventable, or at least recognisable early enough to prevent the bladder from becoming grossly over-distended. It should be looked for in anyone suspected of an obstructed urinary flow, especially after surgery, since the combination of surgery and anaesthetic can cause the bladder not to empty properly.

The same is true of women in labour, where the combination of the baby's head pressing on the urethra and pain-relieving drugs can impede bladder emptying.

VESICOURETERIC REFLUX
In this disorder, urine squirts back up the ureters to the kidneys, against the usual direction of flow.

The problem is that the urine can carry infection into the kidneys, causing recurrent urinary tract infections (UTIs) and kidney scarring. The condition is commonest in children, but if it is not recognised, its effects can last a lifetime.

What are the causes?
The main cause is congenital abnormalities of the urinary system. Sometimes the valve-like arrangement of the ureter entering the bladder is not properly formed, allowing urine to flow back towards the kidneys when the bladder contracts. This is quite common in infancy, but often resolves by adulthood. It is a frequent cause of UTIs in children, and must be investigated. Reflux can develop in later life as the result of an obstructed outflow of urine from the bladder.

What are the symptoms?
There are no direct symptoms of vesicoureteric reflux itself, only of the recurrent UTIs that it causes.

How is it diagnosed?
A micturating cystourethrogram (p. 101) should be considered in all children following their first UTI. A delay in diagnosis will lead to scarring and long-term damage to the kidneys. Up to 60 per cent of children investigated for UTI have vesicoureteric reflux.

What are the treatment options?
Since 80 per cent of cases resolve as the child grows, all that is needed is treatment with continuous low-dose antibiotics to prevent kidney infection and follow-up with regular midstream urine samples (MSU) and scans of the kidneys. If the reflux is severe and kidney scarring continues, surgery to reimplant the ureters in the bladder is considered.

What is the outlook?
Although the condition cannot be prevented, its harmful effects can. Ultrasound scans in pregnancy can allow diagnosis before birth. The earlier it is picked up, the sooner measures can be taken to reduce long-term damage.

Index

Acknowledgments

Carroll & Brown Limited would also like to thank:

Picture researcher
Sandra Schneider

Production manager
Karol Davies

Production controller
Nigel Reed

Computer management
Paul Stradling

Indexer
Jill Dormon

3-D anatomy
Mirashade/Matt Gould

Illustrators
Andy Baker, Rajeev Doshi/Regraphica, Jacey, Kevin Jones Associates, Debbie Maizels, Mikki Rain, Halli Verrinder, John Woodcock

Layout and illustration assistance
Joanna Cameron

Photographers
Jules Selmes, David Murray

Photographic sources
SPL = Science Photo Library

1 GJLP/SPL
6 *(left)* CNRI/SPL
8 *(top)* PH Saada/Eurelios/SPL
   (bottom) Andrew Syred/SPL
10 *(top)* PH Saada/Eurelios/SPL
10–11 Oscar Burriel/SPL
11 Getty Images
12 *(top)* SPL
13 Fuste-Raga, Jerrican/SPL
15 Prof. P Motta/Dept of Anatomy, Rome/SPL
21 CNRI/SPL
23 BSIP Estiot/SPL
26 *(top)* Prof. P Motta/Dept of Anatomy, Rome/SPL
   (bottom) Eye of Science/SPL
33 *(top)* Dr T Blundell. Dept of Crystallography, Birkbeck College/SPL
   (bottom) Biophoto Associates/SPL

34 Ed Reschke, Peter Arnold Inc/SPL
38 Jose luis Pelaez, Inc/Corbis
38–39 *(centre)* Photomanipulation by Nick Veasey/Untitled
39 Getty Images
40 *(left)* Getty Images-Foodpix
   (right) Getty Images
42 *(left)* Getty Images
   (2nd from top Getty Images)
   (3rd from top Getty Images)
44 *(top,bottom)* Getty Images
46–50 Getty Images
54 *(left)* Getty Images
55 *(right)* Getty Images
60 Getty Images
61 *(left)* Getty Images-Foodpix
   (top right, centre) Getty Images
63 Getty Images
64 Getty Images
65 *(left)* Getty Images
66 *(top)* Getty Images-Foodpix
   (centre, centre below, bottom) Getty Images
67 *(top left, top right, centre, bottom)* Getty Images
69 Getty Images-Foodpix
73 *(left)* Getty Images-Foodpix
   (top right) Getty Images
74 Getty Images
79 Getty Images-Foodpix
83 *(left, top right, bottom)* Getty Images
85 Getty Images
86 Getty Images
90 Getty Images
92 *(left)* GJLP/SPL
   (right) CNRI/SPL
93 Chris Priest/SPL
96 Getty Images
99 Saturn Stills/SPL
102 GJLP/SPL
103 *(top)* ISM/SPL
   (bottom) CNRI/SPL
104 *(left)* BSIP, Cavallini James/SPL
   (right) GJLP/SPL
105 Dr Aine Burns, Royal Free Hospital
   (inset) Professor Stephen Powis, Royal Free Hospital
106 *(top)* Alexander Tsiaras/SPL
   (bottom) Will and Deni Mcintyre/SPL
107 CNRI/SPL
108 Getty Images
111 John Greim/SPL
114 Chris Priest/SPL
116 Getty Images

117 *(top)* www.dialysis-cruises.com
   (bottom) Getty Images
119 Alexander Tsiaras/SPL
120 Alexander Tsiaras/SPL
123 Hank Morgan/SPL
124–125 Antonia Reeve/SPL
125 *(bottom right)* Simon Fraser/SPL
127 PH Plailly/Eurelios/SPL
128 CNRI/SPL
130 Mauro Fermariello/SPL
131 Department of Clinical Radiology, Salisbury District Hospital/SPL
132 Hank Morgan/SPL

Back cover *(left)* Eye of Science/SPL
(right) CNRI/SPL

Contact details
NHS Direct 0845 4647
www.nhsdirect.nhs.uk

Information on dialysis cruises:
www.schiffsdialyse.de
www.dialysistravel.com.au

Aquaflex pelvic floor system (photo on p112) available from Aquaflex:
freephone helpline 0808 100 2890
www.aquaflexcones.com

Neen HealthCare
Tel 01362 698966
www.neenhealth.com